Pharmaceutical Project Management

DRUGS AND THE PHARMACEUTICAL SCIENCES

Executive Editor

James Swarbrick
AAI, Inc.
Wilmington, North Carolina

Advisory Board

DRUGS AND THE PHARMACEUTICAL SCIENCES

A Series of Textbooks and Monographs

ADDITIONAL VOLUMES IN PREPARATION

Pharmaceutical Project Management

edited by
Tony Kennedy
Roche Products Ltd.
Welwyn Garden City, England

Marcel Dekker, Inc.   New York · Basel

Library of Congress Cataloging-in-Publication Data

Pharmaceutical project management / edited by Tony Kennedy.
p. cm. -- (Drugs and the pharmaceutical sciences ; 86)
Includes bibliographical references and index.
ISBN 0-8247-0111-9 (alk. paper)
1. Pharmaceutical industry. 2. Industrial project management.
I. Kennedy, Tony.   II. Series: Drugs and the
pharmaceutical sciences; v. 86.
[DNLM: 1. Drug Industry--organization & administration. 2. Drug
Evaluation. 3. Research--organization & administration. W1 DR893B
v.86 1998 / QV 736 P53617 1998]
RS192.P465 1998
615'.19--dc21
DNLM/DLC
for Library of Congress   97-31537
                                                  CIP

This book is printed on acid-free paper.

Headquarters
Marcel Dekker, Inc.
270 Madison Avenue, New York, NY 10016
tel: 212-696-9000; fax: 212-685-4540

World Wide Web
http://www.dekker.com

The publisher offers discounts on this book when ordered in bulk quantities. For more information, write to Special Sales/Professional Marketing at the headquarters address above.

Current printing (last digit):
10 9 8 7 6 5 4 3 2

PRINTED IN THE UNITED STATES OF AMERICA

Preface

Drug development is a high-cost, high-risk, and lengthy enterprise. Most drug companies are actively exploring ways to accelerate and improve their drug development processes. Excellence in drug discovery has long been regarded as a hallmark of successful drug companies. It is increasingly recognized that this alone is not enough and must be coupled with excellence in drug development. The latter capability requires that a high-quality, well-motivated, and well-trained staff is in place, and that development vision is matched with good process and procedure.

Project management plays a pivotal role in achieving and sustaining excellence in drug development. The pharmaceutical industry has been relatively slow to implement project management techniques in comparison with other industries. In the past decade, however, most large drug companies have established project management groups with full-time staff whose professional responsibility is the management and planning of drug development.

Pharmaceutical project management has a broad scope encompassing strategic and operational management of individual projects and of the development portfolio. Within this scope reside challenges and opportunities in the management of information flow, personal and organizational decision making, and risk and opportunity assessment. It includes day-to-day management and motivation of international project teams and management of joint ventures. It covers operational planning, which requires an understanding of the basic principles of networking, scheduling, and critical path analysis. It includes an understanding of intelligent resource management in the face of the high rates of project attrition and conversancy with techniques of steady-state portfolio analysis. Integration of planning for individual projects with the management of the total development resource pool presents particular challenges to most organizations. Some companies have made significant progress in recent years to harness the improved technology in information and planning systems to provide a multiuser distributed planning capability better able to support the project demand and resource supply interface.

Pharmaceutical Project Management highlights a number of topics of key importance to the successful management of contemporary drug development. The contributing authors bring a wealth of development experience drawn from a broad variety of companies to capture the diversity of approaches to project management. The scope of the book includes strategic and operational aspects of the drug development management at both project and portfolio levels. Basic concepts and the practical application of computerized planning techniques are considered. Issues and approaches to successful management of international project teams and for joint ventures are explored. Specific consideration is given to decision making in drug development in the context of management structures that vary significantly between companies. The application of project management to particular development areas is described for clinical trials and manufacturing groups. Also, development work is increasingly contracted out by the pharmaceutical industry, bringing with it specific issues to contractor and contractee. The issues and solutions of both parties are considered.

The audience for this book will most likely include those in drug development and project management, as well as pharmaceutical industry consultants and project managers in other industries, e.g., chemical and food.

Looking to the future, the impact of the dramatic pace of change in information technology on project management is considered. Last but not least, the future role of the professional project manager is discussed, including a review of candidate profile and training needs.

Tony Kennedy

Contents

Contributors

Stephen Allport, C.Biol., D.M.S., Dip.M. Director, Portfolio Planning, Worldwide Project Planning, GlaxoWellcome Research and Development, Greenford, Middlesex, England

Andrew J. M. Black, M.B.B.S. Consultant, Andersen Consulting, London, England

Donald N. Cooper, M.B.A. Global Project Leader, International Project Management, Hoffmann-La Roche, Nutley, New Jersey

David A. Dworaczyk, Ph.D. Director, Worldwide Computer Aided Registration Systems, Research & Development, Solvay Pharmaceuticals, Inc., Marietta, Georgia

Nick Edwards, M.A., B.M.B., B.Ch. Associate Partner, Andersen Consulting, London, England

Helen Grant Consultant, Andersen Consulting, Manchester, England

Tony Kennedy, Ph.D.* Project Director, Project Management Group, SmithKline Beecham Pharmaceuticals, Essex, England

Carl A. Kutzbach, Ph.D.[†] Central Project Management, Pharma Division, Bayer AG, Wuppertal, Germany

Alec MacAndrew, Ph.D. PA Consulting Group, Cambridge Technology Centre, Melbourn, Hertsfordshire, England

Frank R. Mangan, Ph.D. Principal Consultant, F.R.M. Associates Consulting Services, Surrey, England

Ian Reynolds Major Programmes Manager, Logica UK Limited, London, England

Leslie B. Rose, C.Biol., MI.Biol. Managing Director, Medical Scientific Services Ltd., Salisbury, England

Astrid H. Seeberg, Ph.D. Head, International Project Planning, The Bracco Group, Milan, Italy

Stephen R. Self, M.B.A. European Technical Director, Technical Directorate, Merck Generics Ltd., Kent, England

Albert J. Siemens, Ph.D. Executive Vice President, ClinTrials Research, Inc., Research Triangle Park, North Carolina

Ian Trout, C.Eng., M.I.E.E. Manager, Andersen Consulting, Manchester, England

Paul H. Willer, MI.Mech.E., C.Eng. Associate Partner, Andersen Consulting, London, England

---

Current affiliation: Head of Training and Global Team Leader, Project Management, Roche Products Ltd., Welwyn Garden City, England.
[†]Retired.

1

Strategic Project Management at the Project Level

Tony Kennedy*

SmithKline Beecham Pharmaceuticals
Essex, England

I. PROJECT STRATEGY OVERVIEW

Drug development is not a simple process. If honest, most newcomers to drug development will concede that their initial experience as a project team member for a development project is disconcerting. Unfamiliar technical acronyms fly around the room. Team members with greater development experience and knowledge of the project often dominate the discussion. The new team members probably will be glad to conclude their

---

Current affiliation: Roche Products Ltd., Welwyn Garden City, England.

1

contribution to team discussion and to escape from their first team meeting without making fools of themselves. Drug development is more comprehensible if the team member has the good fortune to join a project team at its inception rather than, as is often the case, as a replacement team member. It is at the initial team meetings that the core early development strategy is decided.

Successful drug development depends on the quality of the development strategy. Ultimately, successful drug development is about translating science into an optimal investment proposal that provides value to a variety of stakeholders and customers. This can be achieved only be establishing a strategy which recognizes who the customers for new medicines are and addresses their needs. This will mean moving increasingly from designing "for" to designing "with" the customer. Health care provided in most countries has experienced significant change in recent years. Probably the greatest change to be faced in the future will be the expectation that new medicines will be not only safe and effective but also cost effective in the overall context of disease management.

Drug development strategy is concerned with establishing clearly set objectives for the development and life cycle management of an asset, recognizing critical hurdles to success, and structuring plans to achieve the best reward/risk for the investment. It requires a range of skill sets which include strong technical knowledge of drug development and understanding of development risk management. Project attrition rates are high, and it is important to understand why and when these can occur. The overwhelming majority of projects fail. A primary objective in drug development, therefore, is to eliminate from development, at the earliest time, projects that offer poor prospects for commercial return. Termination decisions are rarely made with certain knowledge which is why they are so often painful for teams and companies to take. It requires understanding of the importance of the target product profile (TPP) as a strategic tool and the need for its continuous review throughout development. The TPP definition is critical to the design of clinical development strategy. It is also the basis for establishing clear Go/No Go criteria for the compound through development.

It depends on good understanding of planning skills to ensure that alternative development scenarios are recognized and their impacts are fully explored. It also requires business skills to evaluate the investment opportunity integrating the key parameters of risk, time, cost, and return. At the core of all of this is knowledge of the disease area which enables the impact of a new medicine in the total scheme of intervening in the disease state to be assessed. If this analysis is at fault, all else is of little value. In an increasingly cost-constrained environment, where cost effectiveness is a passport of access to patient groups, pharmacoeconomics will be a key strategic driver in formulating development plans.

It also requires an understanding of life cycle management. The commercial value of a product will be realized only by ensuring that the product benefits are fully exploited. New medicines will need to "earn their keep" by justifying price at time of market entry and by sustaining their competitive value during their life cycle. An investment in health economics studies will be needed to underpin this case. Opportunities may exist for developing better dosage forms and dose regimens and may also exist for switching Rx medicines to OTC. Finally it is essential to establish a clear postpatent strategy in good time.

In summary many skills are needed to create a strong development strategy. Generally a well-structured project team has these skills. The experienced project manager should have a broad awareness of many of these skill requirements. However, generally, his or her greatest contribution will be in harnessing the skills within the project team to build a robust and farsighted project strategy.

II. DEVELOPMENT STRATEGY FROM CRADLE TO GRAVE

A. Early Development Strategy

1. Improving Input Quality to Development

The quality and quantity of preclinical data provided by discovery groups to support the development of a new compound is often suboptimal. It is important to establish appropriate selection criteria for development because much time and resource can be wasted, subsequently, by the development organization in "patch and mend" strategies which more thought (and training) in discovery could obviate. This is not to advocate a fortress mentality with development playing a prima donna role to discovery. There has to be a reasonable balance with the onus of responsibility on discovery to provide a basic array of technical data to justify development and an onus on development to show maturity and reasonable flexibility. Specific data gaps in a development proposal may exist for good reasons (e.g., obtainable but will incur major delay) and can be addressed in development. Establishing reasonable criteria for development is also valuable to discovery groups though this may not be appreciated at the time! The selection criteria can be used to better discriminate between alternative lead candidates prior to development. Generally, lead candidates are selected on the basis of structural activity studies focused on one or more biological activities. It also makes good sense to optimize development candidate selection by examining other preclinical data which will be critical for development. In each of the nonclinical development disciplines (chemistry, pharmaceutics, drug metabolism, pharmacokinetics and toxicology) key pieces of data may be obtainable at modest cost and to aid in selecting the best development candidate. Basic stability and solubility studies of a drug substance, at an early stage may reveal the need to select a better salt or an alternative candidate. Characterizing the basic pharmacokinetics may highlight a best option candidate. In vitro genotoxicity testing should certainly be undertaken early. Although additional resources are required to more fully profile a limited selection of development lead candidates, the payback in improved input quality to development will more than justify the effort.

2. The Product Profile—A Strategic Tool for Drug Development

The key strategic tool which guides drug development is the Target Product Profile (TPP). The TPP describes the specifications of the product intended to be introduced into the market [1]. It defines the required efficacy and side effect profile of the product, how it is supplied, how it is to be used, in which patient groups, and for what purpose. It specifies the cost of goods and the time of market introduction. It is the key design template for creating the development plan. It defines the performance requirements which enables the commercial organization to assess the market impact and estimate the commercial return. Teams sometimes confuse what they hope to see in the performance of a development compound with the minimum performance that would provide for a viable commercial opportunity. It is essential to define a *minimum* TPP specifying the *minimum* performance for commercial viability. The expected product performance can also be defined alongside the minimum TPP, and commercial forecasts can be provided for both. The specific attributes within the TPP constitute a package. If a change is made in one attribute, the whole TPP must be reviewed again to ensure that the impact of the change is fully understood. The TPP has to be set in a specific time frame for launch because any change in schedule may result in an important change in the market environment, e.g., competitor launch.

The TPP is dynamically affected by internal and external factors. Internal factors can include clinical and nonclinical development findings. External factors include, for example, new competitor clinical results just released. Therefore, the TPP is generally reset in development. The TPP is a contract between R&D and the commercial organization (Fig. 1). The

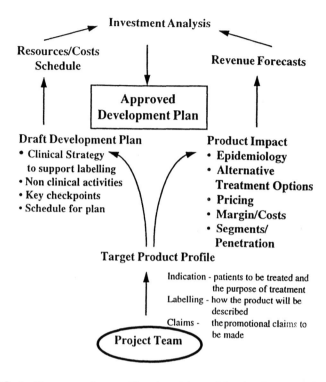

FIG. 1 Target product profile—key driver of the development plan.

development investment is endorsed by the commercial organization on the basis that the TPP specifications are delivered at an agreed time and cost. If the TPP "contract" is to be changed, this must be renegotiated and an endorsement for the new contract secured to ensure that further investment is justified.

The TPP is the pole star on which the development plan is focused. The TPP is valuable only if it is specific and quantitative. The TPP enables setting development checkpoints based on the minimum performance established in the TPP. The TPP should be defined by the project team because it is a multidisciplinary task. To frame the TPP, the team must define how the drug is intended to be used in the disease state. A good start for the project team is to attempt a pictorial (disease cartoon) depiction of the patient flow in a disease. This would highlight how the disease is detected and how the disease progresses both acutely and chronically. The types of invention possible (current and expected) should be assessed including both prophylactic approaches, surgical intervention and drug intervention. The outcomes of intervention and their problems should be considered. This holistic approach takes time (generally this analysis will reveal important information gaps, a need to collect information, and a need to secure external expertise to help understand the treatment context), but its reward is a TPP of substance and not a "jump to conclusion" profile that simply adds 5 percent to an efficacy parameter of what may be an irrelevant competitive product. One benefit for a company in focusing on selected franchise disease areas is that good information bases and good understanding of specific diseases should already be in place with strong links to health care professionals who understand patient needs in these diseases.

3. Target Product Profile—A Hypothetical Case Study: PRIONIX

Usually it is not an easy task for project teams to draft a TPP. The types of issues encountered can best be illustrated in a hypothetical application. A new development candidate has been created for the following TPP analysis. Experts in rheumatic disease are asked to exercise leniency in their scientific scrutiny of the development support data which follows. . . .

PRIONIX is a novel compound that has advanced to development as an antirheumatic drug based on beguiling science not fully understood at a molecular level! It was shown that PRIONIX binds tightly in vitro to a small protein discovered in the joint fluid of patients with rheumatoid arthritis. Binding resulted in reduced cartilage degradation in a human in vitro joint explant system. Evidence from several clinical research studies demonstrated that the protein was a very potent proinflammatory factor and one whose concentration was a reproducible marker of active joint inflammation. Some animal work was done which highlighted limited bioavailability for PRIONIX: oral and IV studies established acceptable acute toxicity and demonstrated no significant issues in pharmacological safety studies. A decision was taken to develop PRIONIX.

The project team drafted the TPP. The key components of the TPP were addressed in defining the indication(s), the dose regimen, the required efficacy, acceptable safety, and tolerability profile. The maximum intended cost of goods was defined, and the time frame to market launch was projected.

Key competitor compounds in development and in the market were reviewed to ensure that the minimum criteria were adequate. The market dynamics in the period following launch were considered in detail to highlight events that could have a significant impact on prescribing the medication.

Such events could include introduction of new diagnostic tools (which might increase or decrease the patient pool), major competitors going off patent with an impact on pricing, and regulatory and market interventions which could restrict use. This analysis identified the major factors which could affect market penetration and commercial success.

In discussing the TPP, it was recognized that, on the basis of the biological data, PRIONIX might offer benefit as an anti-inflammatory agent and as a disease modifying agent or both. The team recognized that the minimum TPP for an anti-inflammatory agent and a disease modifying agent would be very different. PRIONIX could occupy different segments in the market. If the clinical benefit offered was solely anti-inflammatory efficacy, the TPP must identify features differentiating PRIONIX from the best alternative anti-inflammatory drugs currently marketed (NSAIDS) or in development. A review of the literature highlighted that these drugs offered prompt onset of anti-inflammatory and analgesic actions and variable patient response [2] and that some offered a convenient oral once daily dose regimen. It was noted that several agents were already generic and low priced. Important weaknesses were the poor tolerance of NSAIDs and, in particular, the poor gastrointestinal side effect profile. It was suggested by experts that the latter is class related (through modulation of an arachidonic acid cascade). Significant switching in prescribing of NSAIDs was evident, indicating patient dissatisfaction.

The team believed that PRIONIX with its novel mode of action, potentially, could offer key benefits over the NSAID class by providing consistent efficacy and better tolerability. These features were of more than sufficient benefit to the patient to offset a need for once daily oral dosing. The *minimum* competitive TPP chosen by the team would deliver a product with at least as good anti-inflammatory efficacy as NSAIDs but with a slower speed of onset (i.e., one month). The dose regimen was more frequent at t.i.d. than the many o.d./t.i.d. products on the market. However, it was considered that the key benefit of significantly improved GI tolerability provides a real breakthrough for patients and encourages long-term compliance. It was recognized that PRIONIX, in contrast to NSAIDs, probably would not offer benefit in many other nonrheumatoid inflammatory conditions. To crystallize its thinking, the team drafted the labeling statements it intended for PRIONIX. The clinical trials needed to support these labeling statements were carefully reviewed in considering trial size and powering.

Development plans were prepared, which included definition of clinical endpoints and the quantitative performance required. The planning work established that it would take five years to develop PRIONIX to registration.

Phase 3a trials would be powered to demonstrate at least as good efficacy as the selected NSAID comparative drugs with significantly reduced GI side effects. A good commercial opportunity was predicted. An enthusiastic commercial group was already starting to draft promotional copy "PRIONIX - THE FIRST ANTI-INFLAMMATORY YOU WANTED TO STAY ON"....

However, the minimum TPP for a true disease-modifying antirheumatic (DMARD) drug would be very different. The potential patient groups included adult and juvenile rheumatoid arthritis patients. Review of the marketed disease-modifying drugs revealed inconsistent delivery of efficacy and very significant side effects. The toxicities of these drugs resulted in their second-line positioning, and they were generally used only during active disease episodes. Benefit, when seen, was slow in onset. If PRIONIX was a true, disease-modifying agent, which retarded joint destruction, this would be a long awaited treatment breakthrough. In these circumstances, dose regimen convenience would not be critical in the TPP, though an oral disease modifying anti-rheumatic drug was highly desired. An intramuscular route of administration would be acceptable if adequate oral bioavailability did not prove achievable. The drug would likely be dosed even if side effects were evident but, depending on their incidence and severity, could be limited to second-line use with a more limited commercial potential. The team agreed on a minimum TPP for the DMARD. Table 1 compares key features of the minimum TPP for PRIONIX as an anti-inflammatory and as a disease-modifying anti-rheumatic agent.

A development plan was created. It was recognized that demonstrating disease-modifying activity convincingly would require extended clinical studies during which joint erosion would be carefully monitored. Development to the registration point as a DMARD agent would take six and a half years. The commercial group saw a strong opportunity to justify pricing in an area of clearly unmet medical need, where a strong pharmacoeconomics case could be made.

The potential vulnerability of the investment was recognized on two counts. First, this was a project for which heavy investment would be made prior to proof of its DMARD efficacy. Secondly vaccine and other novel anticytokine projects were in development ahead of PRIONIX. The internal research view of these competitor strategies was skeptical—much promised—nothing delivered—and advised that all the other players were long shots—other than PRIONIX!

The team considered the scenarios of PRIONIX as a DMARD with and without acute anti-inflammatory activity. This raised some important

TABLE 1
PRIONIX Target Product Profiles—Comparison of Key Attributes

	PRIONIX	
	As an anti-inflammatory agent	As a disease-modifying anti-rheumatic agent
Indication	For symptomatic relief of the inflammation of rheumatoid arthritis	For treatment of rheumatoid arthritis to reduce symptoms and joint erosion
Efficacy		
• Symptomatic relief—reduce joint inflammation pain, stiffness, and fatigue	Efficacy at least as good as NSAIDs Speed of onset within 4 weeks	N/A
• Joint erosion	N/A	Radiological evidence of joint protection; onset 6–12 months
Safety and tolerance		
• General	Good ADRs profile which supports broad use	ADR profile does not limit to 2° line therapy
• Gastrointestinal –upper and lower GI symptoms –gastric erosions	Incidence of GI intolerance signifi-cantly better than NSAIDs (<5%)	
Drug interactions	N/A	Can be prescribed with commonly used NSAIDs
Dose regimen	Oral tid	Oral tid (want) Intramuscular (must)

issues. First, if acute anti-inflammatory activity was demonstrated would the product be taken to the market as quickly as possible or would the company, first determine if there were DMARD activity before launching and delay filing by 18 months. It was realized that a business analysis involving assessment of costs, project commercial returns, time, and probabilities was needed.

A second issue was the need for acute anti-inflammatory/analgesic cover if PRIONIX possessed only slow onset of DMARD activity. Lack of adverse drug interaction with NSAIDs was considered an important need because comedication with this class could be envisaged. Whether this was a must was felt to depend on the clinical benefit offered by the DMARD and, specifically, if it arrested disease (or, perhaps, limited very slow subsymptomatic creep). Patients dosed early in the disease with PRIONIX might accept temporary mild symptomatic discomfort because they could not take NSAIDs if they knew that their disease would be reliably controlled within a known reasonable time frame.

The types of issues revealed in the PRIONIX TPP example are common in drug development. In many therapeutic areas, there are a hierarchy of clinical benefits that, potentially, can be offered to the patient [2]. The options require careful analysis to select an integrated strategy for first registration and launch and subsequent development. Separating musts and wants and grappling with trade-offs of individual attributes is a challenging exercise [4]. The minimum product profile often gives a product less attractive than the team believes can be delivered and much less attractive than the commercial group would like delivered. The definition of the minimum TPP, however, focuses minds to link product performance to investment justification and leads to sharper checkpoint criteria for project termination. Careful analysis is needed, when multiple indications are options for a drug, to ensure that the best overall integrated strategy is selected.

It makes much sense to interrogate the potential product opportunity by defining the TPP in the discovery phase. First, it may become apparent through technical interrogation of the TPP that the indication being considered is not viable and the program should be closed (or not initiated). Secondly, TPP may profoundly influence the discovery biological studies undertaken and the selection criteria chosen for development. Discovery support activities may be identified to facilitate development of a novel asset. These could include establishing marker assays to support early clinical pharmacodynamic studies.

4. Selection Criteria for Further Development

The minimum TPP created in the development plan should be used to define the checkpoints and Go/No Go criteria for the indication. The criteria chosen should balance realism and rigor. This is easier to say than to do, and some specific comments are appropriate. The data available at early checkpoints will be limited. Dosing will be of short duration. Patient numbers enrolled in studies will be small. Dose regimens will not be optimized, and hence, neither will the efficacy delivered. It is possible that dynamic markers will have been studied rather than the intended clinical endpoints. It is important not to fall into the trap of mindlessly extrapolating required labeling to early checkpoints. This applies particularly to ultimately desired statistical statements for which early trials will not have been powered.

The primary purpose of setting Go/No Go criteria is to provide an answer to the question, Do the data available at this time justify further investment in the project?

For some projects, competitive products may have helped define the hurdle height of the checkpoint. For some pioneer products, demonstration of dose-related activity against selected markers in early studies may be as much as can reasonably be achieved to encourage investment in the next stage of development.

When should the key checkpoint for full development to the market be set? It may be that efficacy is revealed only at the completion of phase 3 scale trials. This could be the case in prophylaxis studies where many patients are enrolled of whom only a small percentage develop a disease condition and contribute the vital efficacy data. In some indications, clinical efficacy can be clearly demonstrated in modestly sized phase 2 trials. When Go/No Go project checkpoints occur and how their criteria are quantified are very much specific to a project. The outcome of Go/No Go checkpoints is not necessarily go or stop. Phase 2 data may reveal that the dose response has not been adequately explored, and phase 1 studies may reveal poor pharmacodynamic results and also suboptimal bioavailability for the formulation studied. In each case, plans can be redesigned to achieve a successful outcome albeit with delay to the project.

5. Back-Up and Follow-Up Strategy

Discovery and development strategy must be closely integrated to ensure success in bringing products to market. Back-up compounds offer no commercial differentiation from the lead compound in development, whereas a follow-up compound does. The high failure rate in development demands a well-planned, back-up strategy. Sometimes this strategy is simply to identify a back-up candidate and await the phone call from development notifying failure of the lead candidate. Some companies adopt more aggressive

All NCEs (n=198)

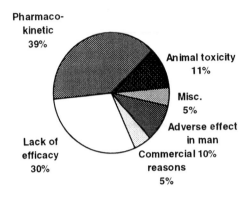

Pharmaco-
kinetic
39%

Animal toxicity
11%

Misc.
5%

Adverse effect
in man

Lack of
efficacy
30%

Commercial 10%
reasons
5%

Excluding Anti-Infectives
(n=121)

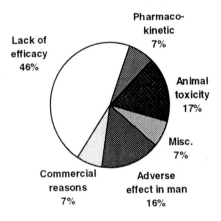

Pharmaco-
kinetic
7%

Lack of
efficacy
46%

Animal
toxicity
17%

Misc.
7%

Commercial
reasons
7%

Adverse
effect in man
16%

FIG. 2   Why do projects fail?

parallel track strategy moving more than one candidate into development from a discovery program to hedge the risk. Does this make sense?

Several factors are worth considering. First, why do projects fail in early development? Some data on this has been published by the Centre for Medicines Research (Ref. [5] and Fig. 2). Anti-infective projects comprised some 77 of the 198 compounds included in this survey and distorted the

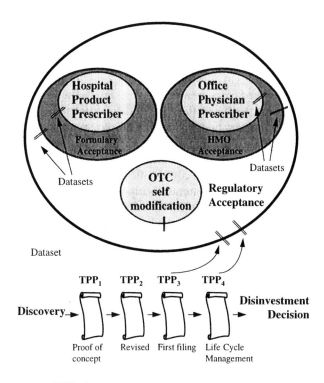

FIG. 3   TPP and data for decision makers.

overall picture because unsatisfactory pharmacokinetics were responsible for nearly all terminations of anti-infectives but accounted for only 7 percent of other categories. If the anti-infective drugs are excluded (Fig. 3 lower panel), by far the major single reason was lack of adequate efficacy (46 percent). Would moving another member from the same series into development address this? This leads to a debate on chemical class, pharmacological class, and idiosyncratic non-class-related effects of drugs. In principle, it might (e.g., better access to the receptor sites, better binding kinetics may be evident within same series candidates). Moreover, toxicology findings, adverse events in humans, and pharmacokinetics together account for 40 percent of the reasons for project terminations. These may have nothing to do with intrinsic pharmacology and may be idiosyncratic. So, in principle, molecular hedging to overcome the reasons for technical failure makes sense.

But there is no such thing as a free meal, and one must also ask how much time is saved by an aggressive parallel track strategy and at what cost. And when would a decision on full development of a lead candidate be taken? The failure rates in development are highest in the early phases and only generically exceed 50 percent in phase 3. But as the chance of success increases during development, the costs of development increase dramatically. So, in general terms, hedging in early development makes sense from a cost/risk perspective. Parallel track development in phase 0 and phase 1 might save 2 years compared with a sequential strategy. The relationships of cost/risk reduction and value contribution for alternative strategies can be modeled. Such modeling, generally, supports parallel early phase development but with a holding rule that a single candidate be advanced for phase 3 development.

In the real world, limited capacities in early development are often totally occupied with drug candidates from alternative discovery programs. The opportunity cost, therefore, has to be considered in a portfolio context where the added value of early parallel lead development may be less than developing lead candidates from other programs. When only one lead is put into development and it is terminated, the delay may mean that a competitive position has been lost. It may be necessary to replace a failed lead not with a follow up rather than a back-up candidate to reestablish a competitive position in development. For this reason, if a company is serious in its intent to establish a market franchise it must sustain a discovery effort focused on follow-up candidates throughout development.

B. Registration and Life-Cycle Development Strategy

Planning in mid-stage and late-stage development has been heavily focused on the first registration of the product with particular emphasis on addressing the regulatory requirements of core markets.

The market for pharmaceutical products has changed significantly in recent times with a broader range of groups now playing key roles in deciding drug usage. This must be reflected in development strategy to ensure that the information needed by key decision makers is available at the right time. Probably the biggest change in recent years has been the impact of cost constraints on health care expenditures which have focused attention on the cost effectiveness of new medicines.

1. Health Economics Strategy

In the past the pharmaceutical industry has viewed the prescribing physician as the key "customer" for a new drug. However, increasingly, the prescribing decision of the physician is circumscribed. Barriers to drugs have arisen in an increasingly cost-conscious health care environment [6]. Although persuaded of the clinical benefit of a new drug, the physician may not be able to prescribe it. Although drug costs per se account for a small proportion (ca. 8 percent) of total health care costs, drug budgets are under strong pressure in most countries. Barriers include national reimbursement agencies, hospital formulary committees, managed health care organizations and national or local agencies with funding responsibilities. These diverse groups will be influenced by data to allow or even recommend using a new drug. The decision criteria and the type of information on which these decisions will be based differ between these groups. An awareness of the different perspectives of the "customers" who ultimately guide drug use is essential (Table 2) to ensure that relevant data is collected to provide a passport of entry (see Fig. 3).

Savings in the drug budget can be made by using cheaper drugs offering equivalent benefit, more effective use of existing drugs, and by limiting access to drugs whose widespread use is unjustified. Cost saving, however, has to be assessed in the broader context of overall health care expenditure. Additional drug cost may well, for example, be easily justified by reduced hospital costs. Demonstrating the cost effectiveness of new medicines will be a critical factor for commercial success in the future. This represents a difficult challenge for the pharmaceutical industry and society because value demonstration is easily supportable as a concept but far from easy to apply in practice. The challenge that health economics poses for those engaged in designing drug development strategy is profound. Many of the real benefits of a new medicine and its true cost effectiveness will not be demonstrable within the scope of clinical trials supporting first registration, pricing, and launch.

An integrated health economics strategy is required that provides data when needed to the relevant customer. In early development, a pharmacoeconomic strategy can be developed with modeling based on epidemiological studies and the way disease management is practiced in the major territories. This will help focus clinical development strategy and highlight the key data sets best demonstrating product value in use. This type of study can be undertaken in phase 1 (or, indeed, earlier as strategic support to the discovery engagement in the disease area). Early development studies should be performed to further define current practices of disease management. This should address the best alternative options of disease intervention and the real-world direct and indirect costs and benefits of such interventions. This work provides a basis for assessing the differential impact of

TABLE 2
Pharmacoeconomics—Interest Groups

Pharmaceutical company	Want an early assessment of project opportunity/ viability; fearful of exclusion of drugs from formularies and HMOs, recognize need to invest in pharmacoeconomic studies but unsure of their impact on decision makers
Pharmacists	Play an important role in deciding which drugs are used in a hospital; this includes formulary decisions and treatment strategy; they help in monitoring patient compliance
Patients	Becoming much better informed and organized in pressure groups increasingly prepared to pressure clinicians and lobby governments; Internet will increase coherence of such groups globally resulting in better attention being given to their needs
Office physicians	Increasingly cost-conscious; generally concerned with long term patient outcome; efficacy focused, they are keen to see time saving benefits (reduced return visits)
Managed case organizations/health insurance companies	Want substantive "real-world" outcome data to select most cost effective drugs; may not have infrastructure to provide this data; not easily impressed with small scale PE studies
Reimbursement agency	Responsible for setting a reimbursement level/co-payment for the drug; concerned with the impact of new medicine on health care expenditures; will set pricing which reflects the perceived cost effectiveness of the new medicine

intervention with a new drug. Therefore, this type of study should be conducted early in development so that its findings are available to shape the pivotal phase 3a study strategy.

Phase 3a clinical studies provide an important opportunity to collect a variety of types of data that can help document cost effectiveness. The limited scale of such trials, the homogenous nature of patients studied, and the protocol limitations do not make such studies typical of subsequent product use. The collection of data for pharmaco-economic purposes in such trials has been described as a piggy-back strategy because the primary driver for such studies is to achieve regulatory approval. The pharmacoeconomics case for a new medicine in a setting more typical of the product in use is better demonstrated in phase 3b studies sometimes termed naturalistic trials. Although, presently, pricing and reimbursement decisions are predominantly driven by nonpharmaco-economic reasons (e.g., competitive pricing, local reimbursement rules), decision makers are increasingly looking for such data to provide a reference range.

With the increasing requirement to justify cost effectiveness, there needs to be continuing investment in pharmacoeconomic studies to sustain justification of product use and pricing. Information technology will facilitate the generation of outcome data from larger population groups in the years following product introduction, enabling recognition of the real product value earlier than previously been possible.

2. Registration and Launch Strategy

The indication selected for first registration and launch of a new product may be one of several that could have been registered. Several factors will generally have been considered in deciding the first registration and launch strategy. These include speed to market, opportunity to set satisfactory pricing in the market, the value of the indication, and coherence with strategy to bring other indications to market at a later stage (Fig. 4). The lead indications for a new drug are generally selected early in development. It is not easy to reengineer filing strategy at a late development stage but development data may necessitate this (e.g., strength of clinical data in different indications). A thorough understanding of regulatory requirements is needed to ensure that trials are designed appropriately to support commercially desired labeling. Where possible, this involves dialogue with regulatory agencies to discuss specific plans. It involves review of relevant guidelines and, for the U.S., review of relevant competitor Summary Basis Of Approval (SBOA) documents. It also requires understanding the attitude of agencies toward particular types of products gained by attending key Advisory Committee meetings. In a number of pioneering areas, regulators and their advisors are struggling to make sense of clinical science just as much as academic and industry specialists. It is essential to be closely attuned to current thinking in such areas and, indeed, for the industry to actively contribute to the debate.

The clinical trial strategy should be reviewed by leading clinical specialists in the major markets in time to ensure that the trials conducted are relevant to the markets and to ensure that opinion leaders are fully familiar

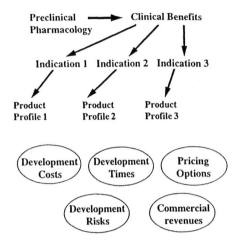

FIG. 4   Indications filing strategy.

with the product and that they, too, can see its value in use. If they cannot, then something is badly amiss.

3. Postfiling and Launch Strategy (Phase 3b/4)

In a number of therapeutic areas, there is often a hierarchy of claims that, potentially, can be registered. In atherosclerosis, shorter term studies may document the effect of a novel lipid lowering agent on systemic lipid profiles, and drugs have been registered with claims based on such data. In longer studies, it may be possible to document that the drug can reduce the rate of progression of atherosclerosis or even better to demonstrate its reversal. Such studies could be done in peripheral vessels or perhaps even more persuasively in cardiac vessels. Still more convincing clinical benefit data could be provided if it can be demonstrated that the incidence of myocardial infarction or stroke is reduced in patients with abnormal lipid profiles. Regulators may wisely not attempt to extrapolate the clinical relevance of documenting different disease-related endpoints but, instead, may grant labeling, specifically, for what has been demonstrated appropriately in pivotal clinical studies. Drugs that are already marketed may have taken up the challenge to mount the hierarchy of claims staircase, creating a major hurdle for new entrants. Indeed, this is the case in a number of therapeutic areas (atherosclerosis, congestive heart failure). A strategic dilemma is to decide, within the scope of development scale clinical trials, whether there is any prospect for demonstrating incremental benefit against "best competitor" claims. It should also be recognized that there is always the possibility that conducting trials to document more fundamental benefits may backfire with disappointing clinical results.

4. Life-Cycle Strategy

Life-cycle strategy is concerned with identifying optimal and coherent approaches to realizing the full value of the asset and translating these into a life-cycle management plan. Adroit life-cycle management can make a major contribution to the scale of the commercial success. The level of risk for investment at this stage is often lower and the return on investment faster than with the earlier development projects.

Life cycle management encompasses

- plans to support the marketed indications:
  The competitive environment continually changes and requires a continuing investment in studies to support the asset. Increasingly, this will be investment in cost effectiveness studies to retain the marketed product in formulary/reimbursement lists or gain access to these.
- plans to extend indications and labeling:
  Frequently there will be opportunities to expand the market by registering the drug for smaller "niche" indications which, of themselves, would not commercially justify development of the drug but add significant value as additional indications. In addition, there may be opportunities to optimize labeling to provide a stronger commercial platform.
- plans for introducing line extensions:
  The first dosage forms and the dose regimen introduced in the market may often be improved on. It may be possible to develop patented dosage forms offering improved pharmacokinetic profiles in humans and providing clinical benefit with reduced dose frequency. It may be possible to introduce more palatable dosage forms. This an area of drug development too easily dismissed as being trivial. This is naive. Convenient dose regimens offer considerable benefit to patients, particularly those on chronic therapy by enhancing compliance and minimizing disturbance to their busy daily lives. Dosing twice a day for children rather than three times a day may be particularly helpful to ensure compliance without the need for medicine to be given at school.

- downstreaming R_x to over-the-counter (OTC) products:
  In some therapeutic areas, it may be appropriate to move R_x drugs to OTC products. There are some obvious merits to this for medicines whose safety has been well established. For conditions which are well self-diagnosed by the patient, availability of the OTC product avoids unnecessary prescribing intervention by the doctor and permits quicker access to the medicine.
- plans for the post patent period:
  Exclusivity is the key factor underpinning the commercial opportunity for a drug. This may derive from a variety of patents on the drug substance itself, process patents on its manufacture, and patents on its use in particular indications and dosage forms. It may also depend on regulatory exclusivity. Commodity market dynamics rapidly follow loss of exclusivity. Decisions will be needed well before patent expiration on whether to compete in the generic market and how this will be implemented. The generic market is a very different market. Taking a Darwinian perspective, the traits that make a drug company a good discoverer, developer, and marketeer of new drugs are not the same traits as those for survival in the generic market. In recognizing this dilemma, some major companies therefore, have set up separate generic subsidiaries.

III. DRUG DEVELOPMENT AS A BUSINESS

Drug development is an investment at risk. The cost of development increases with each development phase. The investment should be reviewed at each key checkpoint in development and should be justified based on the data available.

A. Projects as Investment Opportunities

Drug development requires the investment of substantial money and resources over a significant time period before the launch of the product and the possibility of revenue return. The investment opportunity must be evaluated competently.

Generic probability of success rates at each phase of development are known, and, unless there are very strong project reasons not to do so, generic probabilities should be used (teams *invariably* overestimate the chance of success for their project!) Financial analysis can materially help teams in selecting best strategies by providing a basic pivot of project value around which other project parameters can be rotated.

B. Development Risk Management

It is a salutary fact that most of what we do in development is aborted or completed but never reported. Indeed, in their whole careers in development, many people never work on projects that become products. The impact of attrition is well illustrated in Table 3. This is a steady state portfolio, a mathematical model which has, as its key parameters, the failure rate at each development phase and the time taken in each phase. The model is framed around an objective to bring one new chemical entity to market each year. Based upon the indicated phase durations and failure rates, the portfolio would contain about 22 compounds with most in early development. The failure rate is generically very high in early development. Phase 1 and 2 are particularly severe. It is vital to "cull" weak projects as soon as possible. Such decisions are rarely if ever taken in a state of total certitude. In recent times it has been increasingly recognized that terminating projects is something to be regarded as an achievement, not a failure. Because resource utilization increases considerably at each phase of development, postponement of a termination decision, in effect, wastes resources on a redundant project but costs the organization by denying resources to other projects. Termination decisions are difficult at any development stage but become increasingly difficult in later development because investor expectations are often factored into the company stock price. Portfolio modeling also illustrates the importance of speed in development which is generally discussed in the context of competitor time lines. Faster development also means that a smaller portfolio can sustain a desired product flow with much reduced resource demand.

TABLE 3

Project Failure and the Portfolio (Target—1 NDA per year)

Phase	0	I	II	III	NDA
Input	9	7.5	2.5	1.25	1
Output	7.5	2.5	1.25	1	
Elimination	1.5	5	1.25	0.25	
Elimination rate	1/5	2/3	1/2	1/5	
Phase duration	0.9 yr	1 yr	1.5 yr	1.75 yr	
Chance of NDA	11%	13%	40%	80%	
A goal of 1 NDA per year results in the following steady-state portfolio	8.1	7.5	3.75	2.19	

IV. DRUG DEVELOPMENT INTO THE NEXT MILLENNIUM

There has never been a more exciting time to work in drug development. Dramatic advances in technology will revolutionize the way drugs are discovered. Genomics, robotics, miniaturization, and information technology will synergize to accelerate the pace at which new science is translated into novel drug candidates. The capacity to discover new drug candidates will outstrip development resources. This will accentuate the need for strategic visioning—choosing the best options from the pack to put into development as well as emphasizing, still further, the need to shake out weak projects from the portfolio. Drug development will be particularly exciting because, for the first time in history, our human molecular architecture will be known, revealing multiple vantage points from which to attack disease. Disease management will increasingly be seen in a holistic way by drug developers, drug prescribers, and payers. In so doing, those groups will provide better service to the patient (who was always "holistic"!). Understanding the genetic basis of disease, the availability of diagnostic markers to target and monitor disease states, and the new array of drugs tailored for disease states will transform medical practice. Value assessment of medicines will develop from its present infancy. This will demand a much greater effort to understand the disease state and where a new medicine will make its best impact. Health economics strategy will become firmly embedded in development strategy throughout the development and life-cycle management of a drug.

New strategies will be needed to meet the new challenges presented by new science and new customer expectations. Development strategy will increasingly be set *with* customer groups. Ultimately, it is in the interests of all parties that the true value of a new medicine be revealed as soon as possible, so that all parties can derive maximum benefit. Patients on project teams could rapidly dispel misconceptions about the burden of disease. HMO economists, equally, could rapidly add focus to health economic strategy. An engagement strategy that binds stakeholders and customers together with greater transparency and trust is likely to be the most fruitful avenue for drug development in the new millennium.

REFERENCES

1. A Kennedy, B, Mangham. Project Management in drug development. In: J Lloyd, A Raven, ed. A.C.R.P.I. *Handbook of Clinical Research*. Churchill Medical Communications, 1994, p 364.
2. P S Helliwell, V Wright. Anti-inflammatory drugs. In: J O'Grady and O I Linet, eds. *Early Phase Drug Evaluation in Man*. The MacMillan Press, 1990, p 674.

3. D G Grahame–Smith, J K Aronson. *Oxford Textbook of Clinical Pharmacology and Drug Therapy.* Oxford University Press, 190, p 65.
4. M Corstjens. *Marketing Strategy in the Pharmaceutical Industry.* Chapman and Hall, 1991, p 63.
5. S R Walker, J A Parrish. Innovation and new drug development. In: B C Walker, S R Walker, eds. *Trends and Changes in Drug Research and Development.* Kluwer Academic Publishers, 1988, p 9.
6. E G Feldbaum, M Hughesman. *Healthcare Systems Cost Containment Versus Quality.* Financial Times Business Enterprises, 1993.

2

Strategic Project Management at the Portfolio Level

Stephen Allport

GlaxoWellcome Research and Development
Greenford, Middlesex, England

25

I. INTRODUCTION

Portfolio review and analysis is not new. Techniques have been available and widely used in many industries for a number of years. However, the changes in the pharmaceutical industry and its environment have caused pharmaceutical companies to examine their portfolios with a degree of rigor which, in the past, has not always been considered desirable or necessary. Probability of success must be maximized and cost of failure minimized because future returns are unlikely to allow the industry to cover its risk with the same margins historically achieved. It is becoming increasingly clear that a more structured portfolio review process is required to achieve these aims. The organization will benefit at several levels through

- gaining greater insight into the value of existing and proposed developments.
- gaining insight into strategic issues
- development of analytical processes and tools to assist effective decision making

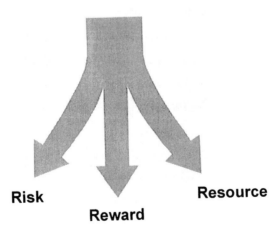

Risk   **Resource**
              Reward

FIG. 1   Three elements to balance in portfolio review and analysis.

• development of a stronger linkage between Research, Development, Marketing and other functions.

Whatever approaches are taken to portfolio review and analysis, the aim is to ensure a balance of three elements, as shown in Fig. 1. Analysis and review of these elements allows the company to determine whether the pipeline is capable of delivering the returns demanded by the corporate strategic aims and ensure that resources are available and directed to those areas most likely to produce future success. The importance attached to each component and the weighting given reflects the individual style and philosophy of the company. Irrespective of differences in style, there are common techniques and processes to provide a robust underpinning to ensure the value of the portfolio review process.

II. WHY BOTHER WITH PORTFOLIO REVIEW AND ANALYSIS?

This section considers the overall value of portfolio review and analysis techniques to the company.

Portfolio review and analysis offers a means to link the strategic goals of the company to its operational plans, as represented in Fig. 2.

Portfolio review forces insight into the value of individual projects and their contribution to corporate aims. It allows optimization of resource usage across therapeutic areas, phases of development, and according to different strategic scenarios.

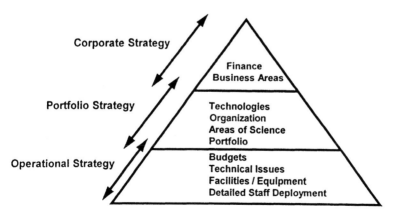

FIG. 2   The link between the strategic goals and operational plans of a company.

III. OVERVIEW OF THE PORTFOLIO
REVIEW PROCESS

This section outlines the key features of the portfolio review and analysis process.
Strategic portfolio review is conceptually very simple:

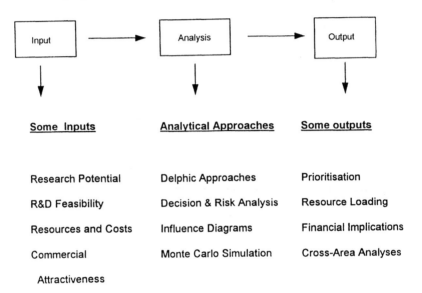

Some Inputs	**Analytical Approaches**	**Some outputs**
Research Potential	Delphic Approaches	Prioritisation
R&D Feasibility	Decision & Risk Analysis	Resource Loading
Resources and Costs	Influence Diagrams	Financial Implications
Commercial	Monte Carlo Simulation	Cross-Area Analyses
Attractiveness		

There is no single "right" method for determining optimum portfolios, but in any successful methodology there is a guiding principle of balance. First, there must be a balance between analytical and Delphic approaches; to some extent this will be dictated by the stage of development of technologies or particular components of the portfolio. In general, the earlier in the process, the less emphasis there will be on quantitative analysis. Secondly, there must be balanced input from R&D and Marketing and from other functions as appropriate. The inputs must be strategic and visionary rather than operational. The third element is the internal/external balance. This applies to environmental analysis and to contribution to the review. A richer and more robust process will usually follow if external, unprejudiced expertise is allied to internal judgment and familiarity with the company, its strengths and its ethos. Fourth, there must be a balance between the time and effort required and the value and credibility of the information obtained for the review.

Although conceptually simple, strategic portfolio review is demanding in terms of information required, but a structured review process will give the organization fresh insights and perspectives on familiar issues.

The cornerstone of the process is the Product Profile. This should be jointly generated by R&D and Commercial groups and should describe the characteristics and features of the product that appears in the marketplace. Key features, such as likely indications, expected therapeutic advantage, advance over gold standard (the best available treatment at the time of launch), and likelihood of reimbursement are included. It also indicates upside and downside potential and the factors which contribute to those positions. The downside profile is usually the minimum acceptable product for the company. Based on the profile, an assessment is made of the likelihood of success and value. Importantly, it recognizes that, ultimately, value is determined only by the customer.

Key considerations are transparency of the process and the need to ensure that the best available knowledge has been incorporated. A wide spectrum of project staff and line managers must be involved to enable this. Responsibilities must be clearly defined, but the aim is to ensure rigorous debate leading to shared understanding between project and line staff and across corporate functions.

Data should be analyzed in various ways to help decision making and to recognize that there are many different portfolios represented by the pool of development projects. It should also be noted that effective portfolio review is a continuous process, not just an exercise conducted annually to feed a strategic plan.

IV. PORTFOLIO REVIEW INPUTS

This section illustrates, in more detail, the key elements which must be considered for each entity under review.

A. Research Potential

The aim is to enable the organization to understand the broad aims of the research being conducted and the likelihood that it is converted to products with the desired profile. Research reviews have traditionally been scientifically focused and conducted through peer review. This process ensures that thinking is not constrained to a narrow therapeutic focus, and it tests scientific rigor throughout the discovery and development process. Its great strengths must be complemented by closely aligning marketing and research without stifling creativity and scientific flair so that there is a shared understanding of the future market and current research endeavors (internal and external) and how they influence each other. Features which must be considered include scientific strengths, the stage of development and robustness of the underlying science, the current level of research competition, and the degree of advance represented by the entity under review.

B. R&D Feasibility

The aim of this assessment is to understand the chances that development(s) under review passes successfully through the development process and delivers a product which meets the desired profile. This assessment is normally undertaken by the experts in each of the disciplines involved based on their knowledge of the compound. Industry and company indexes of historic probability of success provide a starting point for the review but must be utilized with care:

- Most of these historic indices refer to the chances of achieving a registration, not the chances of registering a compound with the desired profile in the markets required at the time required.
- They are historic; newer approaches and technologies will have an impact on their applicability to current methods of drug development. Additionally, few of them yet incorporate the impact of health economic requirements.
- Most are influenced by the traditional customer base of the industry rather than the newer customer groups which have emerged over the last few years.
- Many are consolidations across different therapeutic areas or classes of drug; it must be recognized that there are major differences in the probability of success between, for example, chronic and acute therapies or antibiotics and antidepressants.

C. Resources and Costs

As the cost of development inexorably rises, it is vitally important to factor this into the assessment of the attractiveness of the opportunities available, but particular consideration must be given to the way the output will be used before determining the input information required. In most cases, data on both costs and resources will be required.

Resources are usually estimated in terms of people needed to undertake particular tasks. Questions which might be considered with these data are

- Where are the pinchpoints going to be in the development process? This demands that data are gathered by key discipline together with some feel for interchangeability between disciplines.
- How many people will be required over the time period under review? This requires that consideration is given to the real demands on staff time. Very few are available for 100% of their time because of training, sickness, time spent on administrative tasks, etc. Equally, it must not be forgotten that additional support staff may be required or that attrition has an impact on projected resource demand.

Cost estimation needs equally careful consideration and establishing conventions which fit corporate and legal financial imperatives.

- Many projects give rise to a number of different indications or formulations. Should each of these bear a share of all the development costs, such as initial toxicology and pharmacokinetic studies? One pragmatic approach is to assign all such costs to the first registered indication and to allocate to later indications only those costs which can be directly associated with the additional work involved (particular formulations or clinical trials for example). But this approach potentially disadvantages the first indication to market.
- Similar issues arise in allocating non-R&D costs to projects. Suppose that successful commercialization of a project demands a new manufacturing plant or line. Should the full cost of this be allocated to the project under review or only a proportion assuming that the plant will be used for other products at some time? If the latter, what would be the basis of cost apportionment?
- Project attrition and identification of points at which expenditure becomes committed again must be considered. For example, a clinical trial program may cost $50M over 3 years; the total committed cost at the start of the program is unlikely to be $50M because of staged or progress payments. Ignoring this timing element distorts the real demands for finance.

D. Commercial Attractiveness

The quality of assessing the commercial attractiveness depends critically on the robustness of the product profile. It considers a variety of factors, some highly quantitative others more qualitative. Health Economic issues must be considered throughout the development process. At the later stages of product development, likely market size, market share and reimbursement, and pricing issues are much clearer. Then it is appropriate to give greater weight to more quantitative approaches to valuation of projects, such as Net Present Value and Return on Investment analyses. At earlier stages of development, it is misleading to place too great an emphasis on these features, so surrogates must be found to ensure sound assessment of commercial worth to allow comparison across projects. These surrogates which measure unmet need include assessment of morbidity and mortality, degree of market satisfaction with current treatment approaches, and some assessment of likely customer valuation of the development candidate. Questions for consideration include What is the potential value of the current portfolio? Does it meet corporate growth targets? Is there an appropriate balance of risk and reward? Is activity focused on areas of greatest value for the future?

- Because different methodologies are used at different stages, it is not usually desirable to make comparisons between individual early stage projects and individual later stage projects. This does not preclude comparison between groups of projects, for instance, by therapeutic area.
- Commercial valuation must recognize that there are many different potential portfolios represented by the projects in development. These include different customer groups, for example, general practitioners and specialists, different regional groups, such as developing markets and developed markets, etc. Assessment of the portfolio value varies according to which of these groups is considered.
- Financial evaluation requires agreement on appropriate discount rates. In most circumstances, agreement is easiest when using the company cost of capital. It is important to recognize that this discount rate accounts for financial risk and that the development risk is accounted for by the R&D feasibility assessment. Adjusting the discount rate according to stage of development may lead to double counting for development risk.

V. DATA GATHERING AND REVIEW

This section considers methods for gathering input data.

It is evident that the quality of the process depends entirely on the quality of the input data gathered; all the sophisticated analysis in the world does not compensate for inadequate source data. Several issues must be addressed in deciding how to gather the data:

- the trade-off of simplicity and speed versus quality
- transparency and buy-in across project and line functions
- alignment of expert forecasts with historic precedent.

R&D feasibility data are readily collected by a questionnaire approach which enables a consistency of assessment across projects—provided that the questions are clear and unambiguous. They must relate obviously to the product profile and be easily answered. One approach is to design a series of questions which consider the chances of success at various stages of development with the intention that individual functional experts and Project Teams address their area of expertise. An example is shown in Fig. 3.

In this example, the project team is asked to assess the likelihood of successfully completing each development stage with the desired profile. The team is given some guidance by showing the historic probability of success for the company at this stage. These questions may consider the probability of success at each hurdle in the development process, for example, chance of successfully passing through the research stage, chance of successfully passing through short term toxicology and the associated pharmacokinetic hurdles, chance of successfully completing long term toxicol-

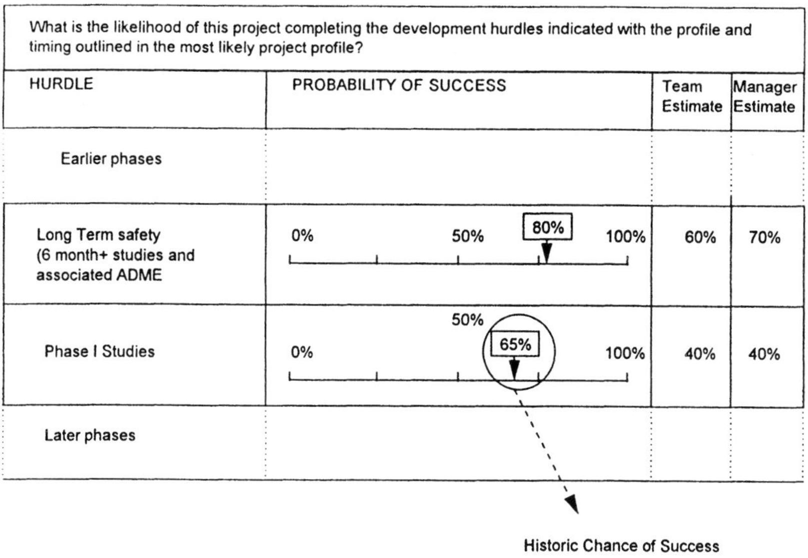

FIG. 3   An example of a chart designed to determine the likelihood of a project successfully meeting intended profile.

ogy and each phase of clinical development, and so forth. Then, the overall probability of success is determined from the product of these individual assessments.

The questionnaire must be designed to ensure that risk factors are not double counted, so it is important to emphasize that each expert should consider the probability of success at that phase, independently of all others.

A second approach is to ask for a single assessment of the overall probability of success. Although this approach has the advantage of greater simplicity, quality is likely to be diminished in two ways. First, thinking may be dominated by one feature which inappropriately colors judgment of the overall value. Secondly, determining probability of success at each key stage allows reviewing the sensitivities of particular projects and the portfolio to each development risk. Thus, if a number of projects are sensitive, for example, to scale up concerns, this may suggest some need for particular attention to that area.

Of paramount importance to successful portfolio review is transparency and buy-in to the source data. In general, project teams generate the source data but these must be reviewed by line management to ensure their support and to take advantage of their knowledge across the portfolio in their area of expertise. It is likely that the project team alone has the necessary in-depth knowledge to understand all the issues on their project, but this must be complemented by line management's ability to look across all the projects and spot inconsistencies or anomalies. This joint approach also ensures full discussion and understanding of assessments to iron out excessive optimism or pessimism.

Commercial and resource/cost data are collected by a similar approach, and an initial assessment generated and agreed to by the project team which may be moderated by line management review.

VI. REVIEW METHODOLOGIES

This sections considers different ways to analyze input data for useful outputs.

There are fundamentally two approaches to reviewing data from the portfolio analysis process. The first is the pure Delphic approach which eschews analysis in favor of debate among experts until a consensus is reached on key issues. The second, this author's preferred approach, favors expert review of data and information derived from a decision analytical approach. The analysis considers probabilities of success, value, and costs.

The most appropriate methodologies vary with the nature of the problem under review, but any method chosen should

- help explore soundness of assumptions
- promote development and assessment of different options
- make explicit implications of each option
- highlight sensitivities of each element
- enable formulation of clear recommendations.

Then, this robust analysis is used to underpin informed expert debate.

There are a huge number of approaches to help give a better understanding of the relationship between the key variables. These include

- influence diagrams and decision trees
- Monte Carlo simulation
- multiattribute analysis
- option pricing analysis.

Each of these techniques takes a structured approach to understanding risk and reward and leads to a consistent view of the likely value of each project to allow a quantitative assessment of its contribution to the total portfolio. It is fundamentally important to understand and manage the risk in the portfolio.

A. Influence Diagrams

Influence diagrams are a visual tool to help understanding the factors which affect the ultimate value of the project; they are a pictorial means of representing a decision tree. Initially, they are used by the project team to ensure a shared understanding of the key issues and how they relate to each other. A simple example is shown in Figure 4.

Each of the important uncertainties, then, is quantified using expert judgment to evaluate the overall impact of risk on return.

B. Decision Trees

Having determined the various factors and influences as outlined in Section VI.A, decisions are made on which courses of action to pursue. Decision trees enable the modeling of risk situations. They are used to determine and display the results of an analysis of probabilities. Each decision may have several possible outcomes with different probabilities of occurrence. Note that the probabilities are multiplicative. Where a number of events are independent, the probability that they all occur is the product of their

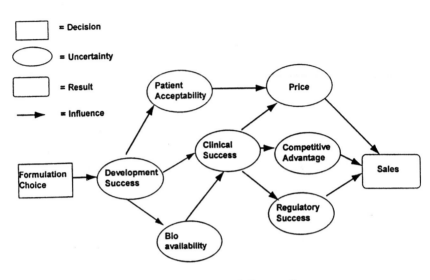

FIG. 4   An example of an influence diagram.

separate probabilities. For example, the probability of throwing two fours with a pair of dice is 1/6 × 1/6 = 1/36. If there are a number of events which are mutually exclusive, the probability that any one of them happens is additive. For example, the probability of throwing either a three or a five with a single die is 1/6 + 1/6 = 1/3. This is important because R&D success depends on all uncertainties being successful. Fig. 5 illustrates the use of a decision tree to show how a decision to invest one of two possible levels of funding into a project affects eventual project value.

In this example, there is a choice of investing either $90M or $50M in a project. Investing $90M reduces overall project risk, but the question is, Does the reduction in risk translate into an overall increase in project value? By constructing a decision tree and mapping the likely outcomes, it is clear that, in this example, the return on the project from investing $90M is significantly higher than the return on the project from investing $50M. Decision trees are the basis of many modeling tools for portfolio analysis.

C. Monte Carlo Simulation

This is a relatively complex technique for risk assessment though there are a number of commercially available software packages to alleviate the

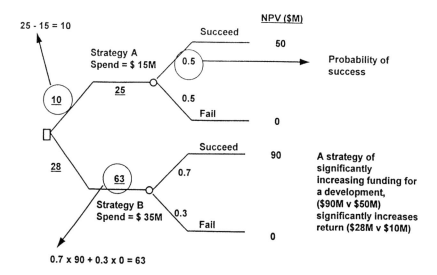

FIG. 5 A decision tree illustrating the effect of investment strategies on eventual project value.

computational burden. The methodology requires that, for each risk in the project, a probability or confidence distribution for the possible outcomes is programmed into a computer. The simulation then takes random values within this banding for each risk and multiplies them together to produce an overall value in the same way as described for decision trees. This analysis is carried out many times with different combinations of values, eventually yielding a distribution of values, as illustrated in Fig. 6.

The advantage of this method is that it clarifies the spread of possible risks and values and shows the most likely outcome and the spread of possible outcomes. In addition to the computing burden, input data generation is much more onerous. It is a technique best reserved either for those companies with exceedingly well-developed risk management capability or specially sensitive situations.

D. Multiattribute Analysis

This is a means to enable evaluation of several options using common criteria. For example, suppose we have two very similar development opportunities with different groups championing each opportunity. We need to

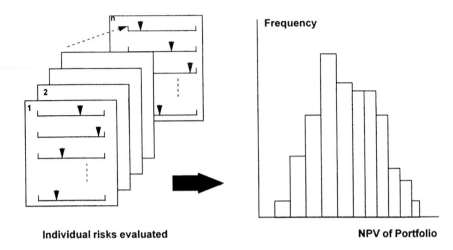

Individual risks evaluated   **NPV of Portfolio**

FIG. 6   A diagrammatic representation of a Monte Carlo simulation.

find a way to build consensus on selection which may precede a more formal risk/reward appraisal or may complement it. The first step is to agree on the key features which the product must have and the key drawbacks which must be avoided. For simplicity, these might include the range of potential indications and launch date as key positives and likely side-effect profile and dosing convenience as negatives. Step two is to agree on the importance of these relative to each other. The third step is to evaluate each of the two options against each criterion to find the preferred option. This process is summarized in Fig. 7.

This is a simple technique, the major strength of which is consensus building based on group preferences.

E. Option Pricing Analysis

This technique has its roots in the financial world. Only relatively recently has its potential in pharmaceutical R&D been considered, though it is not yet widely accepted in that area. The concept is that the drug development process, in reality, is a series of investments based on emerging data. Thus, at each key decision point, the company may choose to continue or discontinue investment. It is not obliged to pay for the full development at the outset, which option pricing values.

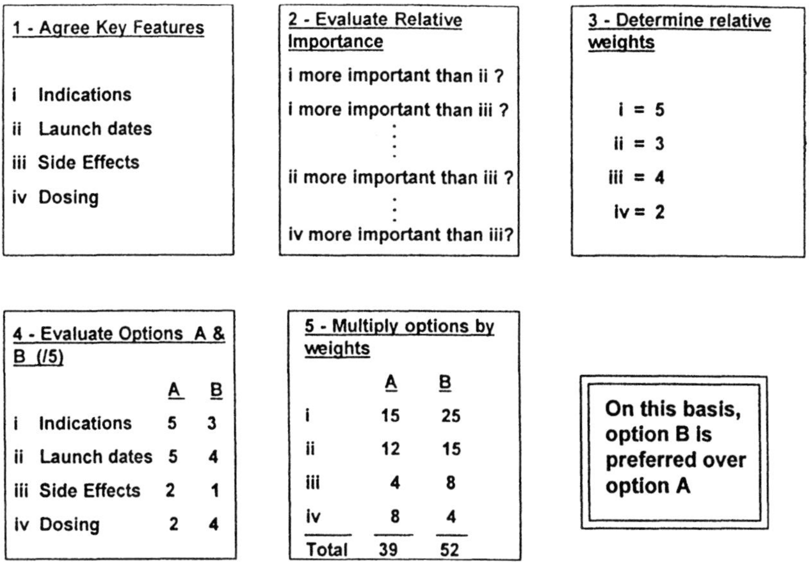

1 - Agree Key Features
i   Indications
ii Launch dates
iii Side Effects
iv Dosing

2 - Evaluate Relative Importance
i more important than ii ?
i more important than iii ?
:
:
ii more important than iii ?
:
iv more important than iii?

3 - Determine relative weights
i = 5
ii = 3
iii = 4
iv = 2

4 - Evaluate Options A & B (/5)	A	B
i Indications	5	3
ii Launch dates	5	4
iii Side Effects	2	1
iv Dosing	2	4

5 - Multiply options by weights	A	B
i	15	25
ii	12	15
iii	4	8
iv	8	4
Total	39	52

> On this basis, option B is preferred over option A

FIG. 7   An example of use of a multiattribute analysis.

This approach is intuitively attractive because it seems to mirror the reality of R&D work. The problem is that the analogy between the financial options market, for which the model was devised, and pharmaceutical R&D is considered unproven by some.

VII. RESULTS

This section suggests some approaches to presenting key portfolio information to enable decision making. In the introduction to this chapter, it was noted that the aim of portfolio review is to balance risk, reward, and resources. These elements should be addressed in the data analysis.

A. Risk/Reward

The most common and readily interpreted output is a simple plot of risk versus return where return is determined by a financial measure such as return on investment (ROI), internal rate of return (IRR) or net present value (NPV). Return may equally be represented by a surrogate for these quantitative measures as described in Section IV.D. Figure 8 provides an illustration of one approach.

This sort of display gives an easy first insight into the portfolio balance with those projects in the upper right quadrant being the most attractive and those in the lower left being the least immediately attractive. If the analysis shows the majority of projects in one quadrant, it may suggest a grossly unbalanced portfolio or a fault in data gathering, review, or analysis. The presentation, however, has limited value. Though it gives a feel for risk/reward balance, it does not assess the degree of financial exposure represented by the distribution of projects nor does it give an easy means of relating the picture to the company's own attitude to risk. Fortunately, this information is added relatively easily.

First, the individual points representing each of the projects can be drawn to show forecast cost or resource demand.

Figure 9 shows the same set of projects as shown in Fig. 8 but redrawn so that the forecast resource utilization over a fixed period is represented by the area of each point. The important lesson is that, though significant numbers of projects appear in the lower portion of the graph, the majority of the resources are allocated to more attractive opportunities. Although this may be intuitively appropriate, it highlights the financial exposure to

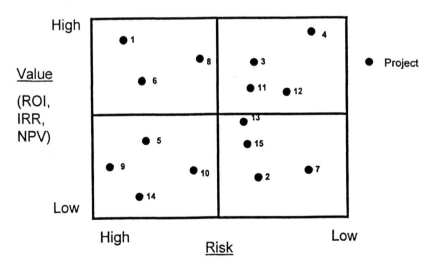

FIG. 8   A display plot of risk versus return.

higher risk projects. It is still not clear from this presentation how the projects can be prioritized in the light of the company's attitude to risk. A further enhancement enables this assessment, as shown in Fig. 10.

The shape of the lines, called isoquants, is determined by the weighting given to the risk components of the review relative to the value components. They allow segmentation of the portfolio into value groups based on the company's own attitude to risk. Vertical lines indicate that, with this analysis, a company is concerned to divide the portfolio only in terms of risk with complete indifference to value. Equally, horizontal lines indicate total indifference to risk and show concern solely with value. In Fig. 10, the shape of the isoquant represents a risk-neutral company that makes decisions on expected value. This could be the complete corporate view on risk or it could indicate, if skewed, that the value data are less robust than the risk data; this might well be the case for the portfolio of early stage projects where reliable market estimates are notoriously difficult to obtain. At later development stages, the shape may be different reflecting an appropriately higher degree of confidence in the commercial forecasts. The important change from Figs. 8 and 9 is that a different group of projects is captured at potentially higher priority reflecting a cut decided by corporate policy rather than the vagaries of a drawing tool.

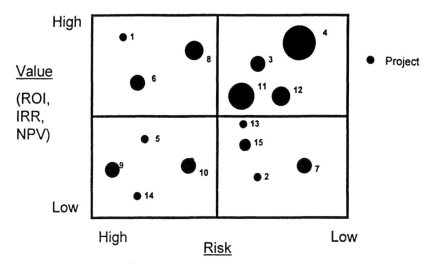

FIG. 9   A display plot as in Fig. 8 enhanced to indicate forecast resource utilization.

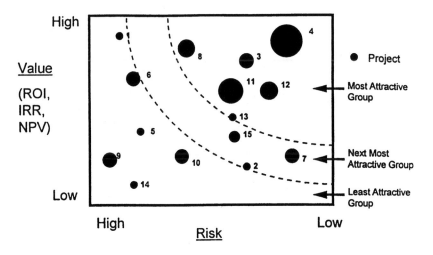

FIG. 10   A display plot as in Fig. 9 enhanced to identify segmentation into value groups based on risk.

It is important to consider NPV and ROI displays separately; they give different information about the projects under review. The former may highlight some projects which look relatively unattractive in terms of overall return, but examination of return on investment may indicate that the projects will pay back many times their investment and would logically be pursued on this basis alone if no other features came into play. Other factors also must be examined to ensure that a balanced picture of the projects under review emerges. Tabulation of the key criteria helps informed review.

	Research potential (max 5)	NPV ($M)	ROI	Chance of success	Strategic fit (max 5)
Project W	5	250	73	50%	2
Project X	3	710	22	10%	3
Project Y	3	75	43	95%	5
Project Z	4	120	62	70%	3

In this example using different projects, on the basis of assessment of overall return, project X would appear highly attractive at $710M, but its risk-adjusted return, $71M ($710 × 10%), is almost exactly the same as project Y with only $75M NPV ($75M × 95% = $71.3M). The latter also has a higher strategic fit value. Looking at return on investment, neither project is as attractive as project W. This brief example clearly illustrates the point that assessing the value of a portfolio in one dimension is misleading and potentially dangerous.

One other key consideration here is the need to compare like with like. Early preclinical projects bear little relationship to late phase III projects in terms of risk profile, cost commitment, or key resources supporting development progression. For these reasons, it is appropriate to group similar projects for comparison, for example, all projects up to phase I or all projects prior to proof of principle. This approach does not preclude comparisons across therapeutic areas or customer segments.

A particularly useful aid to ensuring focus on key issues is examining the sensitivity of the results to different factors. It is relatively easy to look at the sensitivity of any of the criteria contributing to overall project assessment. Consideration of upside and downside values derived from the product profile give a reasonable starting range of sensitivity to be examined. The aim is to ensure that discussion and debate is targeted on the areas which are important and which will impact conclusions. One way to present these data effectively is by a Tornado diagram, as shown in Fig. 11.

This clearly shows that there are major sensitivities around the market entry date and price. The downside of late entry is major, but there is enormous upside potential which suggests that discussion should be focused on how to achieve earlier entry. Similarly attention needs to be paid to bringing down cost of goods—but no time should be wasted debating research potential which has almost no impact on value within the expected range.

B. Resources and Costs

Having considered the risk/reward balance, the next step is to consider resource and cost issues which the proposed prioritization highlights.

Presentation of risk return results, as shown in section VII.A highlights a preferred set of options; appropriate use of the resource and cost data gathered allows determining the resources needed to deliver those options. Figures 9 and 10 indicated how resource demands can be expressed at an overview level. More detail will be needed to help operating managers and project teams. Figure 12 diagrammatically illustrates how cost and resource data simply collected from one source are used to illustrate a variety of key features across the portfolio.

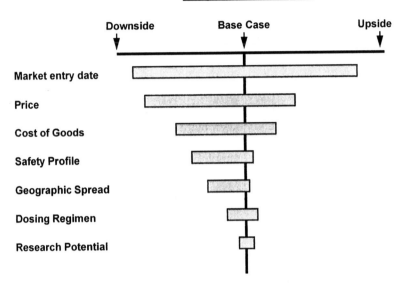

FIG. 11   Example of a tornado diagram.

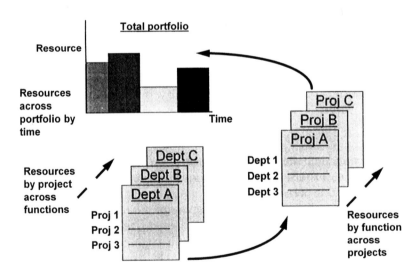

FIG. 12   A diagram showing how cost and resource data illustrate a variety of key features across the portfolio.

Risk-adjusted resource forecasts are required to help line managers define future resource needs and identify potential pinch points. These are usefully supplemented with more detailed information on expected distribution by agreed priority groups. An example is shown in Figure 13.

Figure 13 clearly shows significant increases in resource requirements in Toxicology, Statistics and Clinical in future years. If these are outside expected budget, then the immediate implication is that new staff is required or some contracting-out of work is appropriate. However looking at the second graphic, it is clear that relatively little effort is focused on the highest priority projects. There is obviously scope for reallocating staff; re-iteration of the available risk/return data quickly indicates the implications for return and risk if staff are reallocated.

C. Strategic Issues

The portfolio analysis should provide easily digested data to aid prioritization and understanding and also information to drive future direction. This more strategic view demands considering rather different views of the available data. For example, although Figs. 8–10 provided a view of the overall value of the portfolio, there is no feel for the timing of delivery of that value

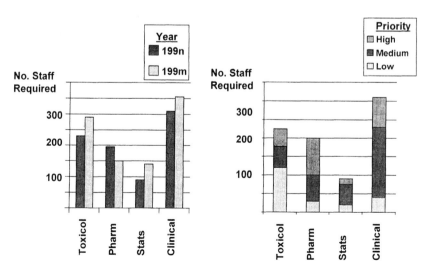

FIG. 13   A risk-adjusted resource forecast distributed by priority groups.

nor of the areas where it will be delivered. Will the portfolio deliver in the short, medium and long term and is the delivery in areas of longer term strategic interest to the company? There are numerous possible questions along these lines. Figure 14 suggests how information to help decisions on these two questions may be presented.

Last in this section, consideration should be given to optimizing the portfolio. There are several tools and approaches available to help this and there are many different optimizations possible. To take one example, through the use of a productivity graph, an "efficient" prioritization may be made, as shown in Fig. 15, which uses the data from the table in section VII.A.

Projects are ordered by a measure of productivity or return on investment using feasibility adjusted revenues and costs. By graphing the cumulative costs and sales, diminishing returns can be observed. In this way, the effect of constrained resources on sales is determined. Although the projects furthest to the right have the lowest priority using this measure, they may also have other qualities that make them attractive. In reality, some projects with low returns will continue to be pursued because of outstanding medical need, regulatory imperatives or other demands which override pure financial concerns. They may also, as in this example, be attractive for their net

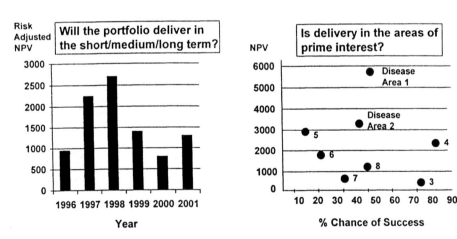

FIG. 14   A graphic presentation to illustrate results versus time (left panel) and strategic interest (right panel).

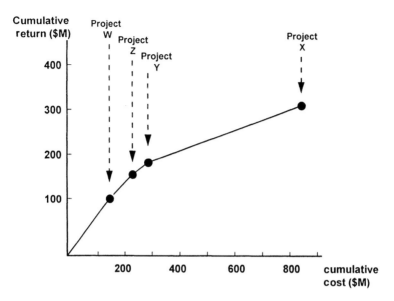

FIG. 15 Example of use of a productivity graph to help prioritization.

earnings. This is addressed directly through an optimization method called integer programming.

Integer programming has not been used extensively with portfolio management. However, it does have the potential to help determine the greatest value of the portfolio with given resource constraints. An objective such as "maximize return (i.e., sales minus costs)" is programmed with a preestablished resource limit. The program determines the mix of projects that produces the highest return. In this example, if resources were just short of $800M, an integer programming solution suggests dropping project Y, even though it has a better return on investment than project X. In a large, complex portfolio, the optimal mix may not be so obvious.

VIII. ORGANIZATIONAL ISSUES

This section explores the cultural and organizational concerns raised by implementing a portfolio review process.

Successful portfolio review poses a number of organizational challenges. Key issues include

- transparency and involvement of all levels of the organization
- open communication of sensitive information
- clarity of roles and responsibilities
- management of the impact of prioritization.

High-quality input to the process is achieved only with staff involvement at all organizational levels, with free sharing of information, and open debate. Project team members must be prepared for their views to be challenged by line management, and line management must equally accept challenge of their views which may be seen to undermine their traditional authority. Reasons for reaching conclusions must be open. In this way the strength of diversity is harnessed to enhance the overall quality of assessments.

Portfolio review requires presentation and sharing of information which may be sensitive internally and externally. Management of information needs to be built into the review process to ensure that internal concerns or expectations are not unduly raised or dashed and that information which may impact share price is not released in an uncontrolled fashion.

Although the need for balanced and broad input to the process is essential and the aim is to build consensus, some group or individual must take responsibility for each element of the process. For example, if project teams develop a series of assessments of chances of technical success, and line management disagrees, whose views should prevail? Each company must decide based on its own culture and approach to matrix management.

A key output of the portfolio review process is prioritization of individual projects. Two important considerations must be borne in mind. The first is to ensure that there is a clear, organizationwide understanding of different categories of priority. Does "high" priority mean that, in every circumstance, these projects will command unlimited resources? Does "low" priority mean that the projects will progress only if there is nothing else to do? Clarity of understanding is essential. Secondly the psychological impact of grading a project as less than "high" priority should not be underestimated—particularly if the project previously had high priority. Procedures need to be put into place to ensure that project teams and leaders remain motivated and committed and that the organizational behavior recognizes that any projects remaining in the portfolio after a rigorous analytical process are valuable and need to be pursued with vigor.

Last, management must reinforce the output with appropriate behavior. If recommendations are not followed with decisive and sometimes painful action, the exercise is seen as futile.

IX. CONCLUSIONS

The pharmaceutical market is changing rapidly and we may not yet know how it will look in a few years time. Portfolio Analysis is a tool to help ensure that companies are positioned to meet these challenges with greater confidence. Effective use of these tools

- provides an agreed representation of the attractiveness of areas of research or development candidates
- defines portfolio gaps and licensing opportunities
- helps understand and manage risk
- helps identify and get rid of losers early
- improves decision quality
- dissolves functional barriers while enhancing respect for individual specialisms.

ACKNOWLEDGMENTS

I am indebted to my colleagues Stuart Harris and Andy Seamans at GlaxoWellcome for their constructive and helpful advice in preparing this chapter.

3

Project Planning
From Basic Concepts to Systems Application

Carl A. Kutzbach*

Bayer AG, Wuppertal, Germany

---

*Retired.

I. INTRODUCTION

A. What Is Planning?

Planning is the process of producing a plan. A good plan optimizes the process to achieve the target objectives of the project in the shortest possible time with the minimum resources. Planning, therefore, means optimizing the classical project management triangle Performance/Time/Cost.

In addition, a plan is an essential means of communication between all project participants to achieve transparency, understanding, and commitment. "Planning makes you free" seems to be a contradiction, but, in reality, the efforts devoted to creating a good plan provide the reassurance and freedom of mind that everything that reasonably could be anticipated has been thought of and considered. Of course, unexpected events occur and make it necessary to review and adapt even the best prepared plan.

A plan for developing a drug gives answers to three questions:

What program of experiments and studies need to be conducted and reported to reach the targeted project performance?
What is the minimum time required to execute this program?
What resources are required to carry out the work and what is the schedule?

This article will focus on the aspects of performance and time planning. Time optimization planning should assume, initially, that resources are available as and when needed. In a second step it may be necessary to adapt a plan to available resources and existing priorities.

The planning targets of high performance and short development time present a practical conflict. Performance is defined by the quality of the database to ensure rapid and broad registration approval and good positioning in the market. Adding more and larger studies to improve this performance inevitably adds to the time. Late market entry jeopardizes the commercial return because of shorter patent protection and increased risk of an earlier market entry by a competitor with a similar product. A short time to regulatory submission, however, is worthless if approval failure follows or if commercialization is compromised resulting in the need to add studies during the approval process. Planning, therefore, must carefully define the minimum program to achieve the target without unacceptable risk and, then, must minimize the time to complete this program.

B. Differences of Planning in Research and Development

The development of a new therapeutic drug runs through two major phases:

the research phase of selecting a suitable drug candidate from a large number of compounds screened for activity in vitro or in animal models and

the development phase in which a single compound is carried through the necessary nonclinical and clinical trials required to prove its efficacy and safety and to obtain regulatory approval.

During the research phase the plans for synthesizing new compounds are constantly adapted to the outcome of the screening assays. Long-term planning in this phase, therefore, is largely restricted to the overall scope of time and resources applied to the project. The work is done by a small team focused on the disciplines of chemistry and experimental biology.

In the development phase, however, the contributions of many disciplines must be closely coordinated to minimize the time to interim decision points and to the final project completion. This article will focus on the planning of development projects. Planning is facilitated by the fact that regulatory guidelines and directives are often available to help in designing the development program for a particular disease indication. Generally, development is structured in the phases shown in Table 1.

Planning of the development process is essentially a stepwise, continuous process starting with a defined target and ending with a detailed plan for action. The plan will be continuously adapted in the light of development findings and changing circumstances as shown in Table 2.

II. THE BASIS OF THE PROJECT PLAN

A. Defining the Project Target

Each plan describes the route to a target. A good plan requires and helps to clarify an exact definition of the target. The general target of drug development is an approved and commercially successful drug product. Drug performance targets are commonly described by target indication and route of administration. This is further specified in terms of efficacy, safety, and patient convenience parameters. Parameters, such as socioeconomic benefit, unique selling proposition, and maximum cost of goods may be added. Early in the development process, some companies use draft PI-sheets covering most of these parameters. Others start with a less detailed Target

TABLE 1

Standard Phases of Drug Development

Phase	Start	Main tasks	End	Average duration, months	Average chance of success, %
Preclinical	Development decision	Safety evaluation in animals; pilot plant scale production process; formulation for phase I	Approval to treat first human subject	15	55
I	Start of first tolerability and kinetic study in humans	Safety, tolerability and kinetics in humans; extended toxicology; formulation for phase II	Approval to start first therapeutic study	12	75
II	Start of first therapeutic study	First proof of therapeutic efficacy; determination of effective dose; longer term toxicology	Approval to start large pivotal therapeutic studies	24	50
III	Start of first large pivotal study	Statistical proof of efficacy and safety in a large, diverse patient population; documentation of all results; process optimization and scale up	Completion of documentation for regulatory submission	30	70
Approval	Submission in first country	Response to questions and requests of regulatory authorities; production of launch supplies; pre-marketing and sales force training	Marketing approval	12–48	90

TABLE 2

Steps in the Planning Process

1. Defining the target
2. List of necessary work packages (studies)
3. Determine logical sequence and estimate durations
4. Determine critical path
5. Optimize plan to reduce critical path length
6. Plan resources and adjust for resource constraints and priorities
7. Adjust plan during execution to new data as required

Product Profile (sometimes also called Project Target Profile or similar). In any case, it is essential that the efficacy and safety parameters are defined as quantitatively as possible so that they can serve as design parameters for clinical studies. Of course, the minimum requirements must describe a product that has a good chance to be competitive when entering the market several years in the future. If these minimum requirements are not met in the study program, then, discontinuation of the project must be considered (see example of a Target Product Profile in Fig. 1).

Often a development candidate offers the opportunity for development in more than one therapeutic indication or in different formulations. These form different subprojects which require their own fully detailed target profiles. Before starting the planning process, it must be decided which subproject or subprojects should be developed initially and in parallel and which are taken as options for later additions or line extensions. A parallel development of all possible options, in most cases, would require too many resources and increase considerably the development time to first marketing approval. The selection of the target for the first development may be based on the chance for clinical success, on an expected shorter time to market, or on other valid reasons. Parallel development of two indications is made easier if they use the same formulation and, therefore, can use the same nonclinical and phase I program. On the other hand, the potential of consecutive or combination therapy by i.v. and oral routes may be important enough to justify its parallel development, e.g., with certain antibiotics.

If broad international registration and marketing are intended, it must also be investigated if identical targets are appropriate in all countries or regions. There are significant differences in medical practice, definition of indications, and acceptance of application routes by the patient in different

Project Target Profile

Date:

Project: AZ 1000
Indication: Hypertension

Formulation: **Tablet**

Product Attributes		Realization		
All attributes are minimum requirements	quan-titative	cer-tain	pro-bable	not clear
1. Efficacy				
* Significant responder rate (long-term treatment)	> 60 %	★		
* Dose dependant efficacy		★		
* One well-tolerated dose should reduce diastolic blood		★		
pressure at trough compared to placebo by	> 8 mm Hg			
2. Tolerability				
* Risk/benefit ratio and incidence of adverse events				
at least comparable to ACEIs or Ca antagonists e.g.:				★
metabolically neutral				
no narrow therapeutic index		★		
no negative effects on electrolyte balance		★		
no restrictions when combined with common drugs,				★
particularly CV and MD		★		
no major contraindications		★		
no CNS side effects				
* (a) in contrast to Ca antagonists no clinically relevant				
peripheral edema or increase in heart rate				
* (b) in contrast to ACE inhibitors no negative impact on				
lung (particularly no cough induction) and those renal				
conditions negatively affected by ACE inhibitors				
3. Convenience				
* Once-a-day application		★	★	
* Small, easy to swallow oral formulation				
4. Innovation (USP)				
* Demonstration of 2a) or 2b) without additional adverse				★
effect				

FIG. 1   Example of a possible format for a Project Target Profile.

regions to be taken into account. The intent must be to cover as much as possible with a shared core program and add studies for specific local requirements where unavoidable.

B. Legal and Regulatory Requirements

The plan must also take into account government laws, guidelines, and points to consider of the regulatory authorities in the target countries as well as rules of ethical committees or IRBs. If clear guidelines do not exist, it is useful to obtain the advice of opinion leaders in the field, e.g., on choosing therapeutic targets and clinical endpoints. Furthermore, every opportunity to present the plan to a regulatory authority should be taken to obtain its opinion or consent.

III. PREPARING THE PROJECT PLAN

A. Elements of a Project Plan

The basic building block of any project plan is the single task leading to a defined result. This is commonly called a work package. The defined result, in most cases, is a study report required for IND or NDA submission. It may, however, also be a development or marketing plan or a produced and released batch of drug substance or formulation. For many work packages in drug development, the scope of study and content of the report are clearly defined by regulatory guidelines or by internal company standards. A list of all work packages and their definitions is an essential prerequisite for a standard plan. In addition, the department involved in carrying out the work should be specified. If several departments contribute to a single work package, the responsible department should be identified. There should also be a standard time estimate for executing the work package in the absence of resource constraints and abnormal technical problems.

Often, it is useful to break larger work packages down into smaller tasks, commonly called jobs. Again, each such job must have a defined end point. A simple example is a sequence such as a protocol design, treatment period, data, evaluation report in clinical or toxicological studies. Other job structures may be more complex, such as the many individual experimental studies comprising the technical or analytical IND or NDA documentation packages for a drug substance or a drug product. A list of jobs for each work package serves as a checklist and adds to the definition of the work package.

There is considerable flexibility in defining larger or smaller work packages and jobs within these definitions. Two general rules may be useful for practical planning:

1. Work packages should, preferably, be carried out within a single department.
2. Work packages identify the detail level of planning and time tracking by the project manager, whereas jobs are tracked within the departments responsible for the work package.

Using these definitions, the size of work packages may vary in different companies depending on the agreed distribution of project tracking responsibility between project management and line functions. Nevertheless, some common practices have evolved and a typical project plan contains between 200 and 300 work packages.

For upper management presentation and review, a plan containing all work packages is much too detailed and needs focusing by aggregation. A first level of aggregation may be the combination of individual studies in one discipline into a super work package for each phase, such as all toxicological or animal pharmacokinetic studies in preclinical, the basic clinical phase I program, or all clinical studies in phases II and III. The most condensed plan for practical use is obtained by aggregating all activities into the standard development phases. An example of the different detail levels of planning is given in Fig. 2.

The project plan should also be structured by using defined decision points and milestones. Decision points indicate the requirement of a management decision for continuation of the project. The decision is typically based on an evaluation of completed studies, a commercial evaluation of the project, and a plan covering at least the next project phase. The scope and level of detail of these decision prerequisites must be carefully defined. Milestones are easily measurable time points of project progress. They serve for planning and comparison of progress to plan. A set of practical milestones and decision points is given in Table 3.

B. The First Plan

Generally, conceptual planning should be done from the end to the beginning, starting with the outline of the pivotal clinical trials necessary for approval and, then, adding the nonclinical, clinical dose-finding and clinical pharmacology studies prerequisite to enter the large and final studies. The initial preclinical development phase, however, typically follows a fairly

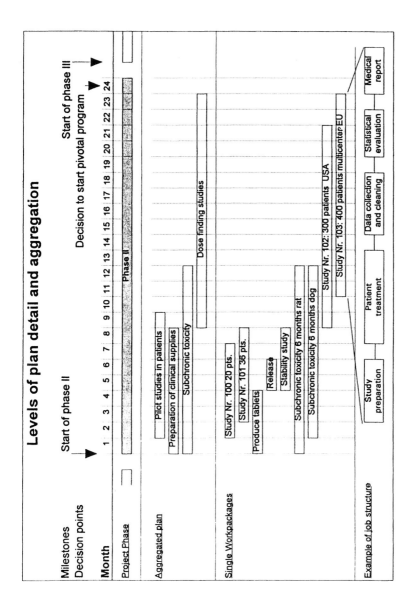

FIG. 2 Example of plan presentations in increasing levels of detail.

TABLE 3
Proposal of Milestones and Decision Points

Milestones	Project phase	Decision to
1: Project presentation	Preclinical	1: Start development
2: Application for IND		2: Start clinical trials
3: Start phase I	Phase I	
4: Start phase II	Phase II	
		3: Start pivotal program
5: Start phase III	Phase III	
6: Clinical cut-off		4: Submit for approval
7: Submission NDA	Approval	
8: Approval NDA		5: Launch
	Prelaunch	
9: Launch		

TABLE 4
Tasks in Preclinical Development

Safety evaluation	
Toxicology	Multiple dose oral or i.v. studies on one rodent and one other species of 2 weeks' to 3 months' duration Mutagenicity tests Reproduction toxicology
Safety pharmacology	Effects on hematology, hemodynamics, respiratory, gastrointestinal, and CNS systems
Pharmacokinetics	Basic kinetics and single dose ADME in two species; autoradiographic distribution pattern; protein binding Metabolism in vitro; toxicokinetics
Production	
Drug substance scale-up	Scale-up from laboratory to pilot scale to produce necessary amounts for phase I under GMP conditions; last chemical conversion step should preferably be finalized
Formulation development	Formulation with suitable stability and acceptable bioavailability for phase I studies

standardized path and therefore, may be planned and started before a complete project plan has been finalized. The main tasks of the preclinical program are shown in Table 4. The early development will be designed after careful review of the preclinical research data. Furthermore, the intended therapeutic use is taken into account for finalizing the toxicological study plan with regard to choice of species and treatment duration.

The first outline of the project plan will usually be a list of nonclinical and clinical studies with their estimated durations and logical dependencies (see example in Table 5). A simple graphical representation of these data will show which sequence of activities determines the critical path of the project and its minimum total duration (Fig. 3). Then, milestones and decision points are added on the time axis. A standard plan is a very useful tool for the project manager to check for the completeness of this first plan and to obtain initial time estimates. However, these must be confirmed later or adjusted depending on resource availability and agreement with the group carrying out the task.

It is advantageous to complement the list and time schedule with a narrative describing the assumptions and rationale underlying the plan. In particular, this should refer to the guidelines and regulations considered. The narrative should also point out which plan details are considered preliminary and need further information for finalizing. It may also be useful to document the reasons for major deviations from the standard plan.

C. Optimizing the Plan

The first plan may result in an unacceptably long total development time. Probably, possibilities of parallel work and overlap have not yet been carefully investigated. In other parts, it may also be too optimistic because some prerequisites were overlooked or do not agree with current regulations.

Consequently, plan optimization above all, should address the completeness of the plan and shortening of the critical path. Effective plan optimization is greatly facilitated by an experienced project manager. He must ask the right questions and insist on a thorough evaluation of the optimization potential. Although safety and ethical reasons prescribe a consecutive and stepwise performance of preclinical and clinical studies, considerable flexibility for optimization exists. Much of the potential for time reduction is in the evaluation phase of studies. However, it is often not necessary to evaluate all data before the decision to start the next study. The following are examples of typical questions to be addressed in plan optimization:

TABLE 5
Essential Elements of a First Plan

Study description	Comment	Result required for item	Estimated duration, months
1. Clinical studies			
1.1. Basic phase I studies	Basic tolerability and kinetics in increasing single and multiple doses	1.3.	6
1.2. Extended phase I studies	Interaction, bioequivalence, special patient groups	1.5., 8.2.	12
1.3. Efficacy pilot studies	If necessary; may be pharmacodynamic studies in 1.1.	1.4.	8
1.4. Dose finding studies (phase II)	E.g., two studies @ 300 patients 2 months treatment	1.5.	18
1.5. Pivotal phase III efficacy studies	E.g., three studies @ 500 patients 3 months treatment	8.2.	30
1.6. Long-term safety studies	Number of patients and duration according to guidelines	8.2.	30
1.7. Special studies	Depending on therapy class and marketing requirements	8.2.	6–24
2. Toxicological studies			
2.1. Acute toxicity	2–4 weeks in two species	1.1.	2
2.2. Subacute toxicity	3 months in two species	1.1.	3
2.3. Subchronic toxicity	6–12 months in two species	8.2.	12–18
2.4. Chronic toxicity		8.2.	12–18
2.5. Reproduction studies	Embryotoxicity first species	1.1.	
	Fertility, embryotox. 2nd species, perinatal toxicity	1.5.	12
2.6. Cancerogenicity	24 months in mice and rats	8.2	30–48
2.7. Mutagenicity	Selection from several in vitro and in vivo tests	1.1 to 1.4.	3
3. Pharmacokinetic studies			
3.1. Prephase I package	E.g., basic kinetics two species, single dose ADME two sp.; autoradiographic distribution, metabolism in vitro; protein binding	1.1.	6–10

3.2. Extended studies	E.g., repeated dose ADME, placental transfer, metabolism in vivo, excretion into milk, entero-hepatic circulation in rat and one nonrodent	1.5. to 8.2. (earlier in Japan)	12
4. Safety pharmacology			
4.1. Basic studies on all systems		1.1.	5
4.2. Extended studies	E.g., safety pharmacology of metabolites	8.2.	6–12
5. Drug substance manufacturing			
5.1. GLP laboratory process		6.1.	6
5.2. GLP pilot plant process		6.1.	6
5.3. GMP pilot plant process		6.2.	6
5.4. Final process	Optimized and validated production scale process	6.5., 8.2.	12–24
6. Drug product manufacturing process			
6.1. Preclinical formulation		2.1.–2.6.	3
6.2. Phase I formulation	A solution may initially be sufficient	1.1.	6
6.3. Phase II formulation	Should have bioavailability of final formulation	1.4.	6–12
6.4. Final (phase III) formulation		1.5.	6–24
6.5. Formulation scale-up and validation		8.2.	12–24
7. Analytical			
7.1. Substance characterization	Including method development	8.1., 8.2.	6–12
7.2. Formulation characterization	Including method development	8.1., 8.2.	6–12
7.3. Stability of drug substance		8.1., 8.2.	≥ 12
7.4. Stability of clinical formulation	Sufficient to support length of study	8.1., 8.2.	≥ 12
7.5. Stability of final formulation	Sufficient to support intended shelf life	8.1., 8.2.	≥ 24
8. Regulatory			
8.1. Clinical trials submission (IND)		1.1.	1
8.2. Marketing approval submission (NDA)			3

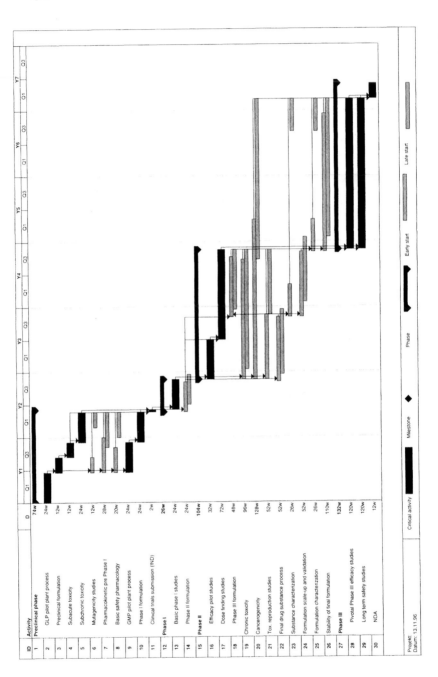

FIG. 3 First project plan drawn as Gantt chart showing critical path and buffer times for noncritical activities (prepared using

a. Completeness of Plan

Have all relevant guidelines been identified and their content been considered?

Do the studies address all product performance statements of the Target Product Profile?

Have all local requirements for the target countries been investigated and considered?

Have marketing requirements been defined and incorporated?

Have all necessary data and qualitative and quantitative material prerequisites for each study been planned with sufficient lead time?

b. Shortening of the Critical Path

Are all work packages on the critical path essential for the start of their successors or can some be completed independently?

What is the minimum output of each critical path study before its successor can be started?

e.g., What length of toxicological exposure is necessary before the start of Phase I?

What part of Phase I studies must be completed before starting the first phase II study?

Can phase III be started based on an interim analysis of phase II studies, rather than waiting for their final evaluation?

What stability-supported shelf life of the formulation is needed before the start of a particular study?

Where are final quality checked reports necessary for continuing the project and where is a draft report sufficient?

How can the study evaluation be expedited, e.g., by concurrent or remote data entry?

Is it possible to increase the assumed patient enrollment rate to reduce the treatment time of a study?

Which task is likely to overrun the estimated duration because of unexpected technical problems and can this risk be reduced by adding resources early?

In the optimization phase, standard duration estimates for work packages are replaced by realistic calendar start and finish dates. Now, the activities to be carried out by development departments can be scheduled with reasonable reliability for the following 1–2 year time frame. If resources in the required time window are limited, the possibilities of adding resources or of external contracting should be considered early.

Published benchmarks of development phase durations can serve as a measure to indicate whether the time lines of a plan are aggressive or comfortable. Real development times show wide variations. Some of this is caused by different study requirements for different indications or by particular experimental or technical problems with the development compound. However, some companies show consistently shorter development times than others, which is probably indicative of good project planning and management. Table 6 lists some recent benchmark data from various sources. An aggressive development plan must aim for a duration at the lower end of this list because the durations shown in Table 6, in many cases, reflect delays resulting from unexpected problems which always occur in practice.

Additional time-saving possibilities may be achieved by reviewing national requirements for technical and safety data or finalized vs. summary reports for clinical trial permissions and placement of studies in territories where these can be expedited. Typically, phase I may be started earlier in many European countries than in the U.S. In contrast, toxicology coverage requirements for phase II studies are less stringent in the U.S. Another interesting possibility is to use the cold season in the Southern Hemisphere for an anti-infective study instead of waiting for the next winter in the North.

The following sections are further practical examples of the necessary considerations and decisions for different tasks of the development process.

1. Toxicology and Safety Investigations

Existing guidelines allow considerable flexibility in designing the toxicological program with regard to species selection, duration, and sequence of studies. The ideal species are those in which pharmacokinetics and metabolism are most similar to the human. Unfortunately, human data are

TABLE 6

Reported Clinical Development Phase Durations for Compounds in Development for Chronic Indications During 1990–1992 in Months

	Europe			Japan			USA		
	Range	Mean	n	Range	Mean	n	Range	Mean	n
Phase I	6–26	15	14	6–13	12	5	6–20	11.5	8
Phase II	12–40	27	13	21–37	28	5	12–60	24	8
Phase III	21–76	38	10	24–73	32	5	28–48	34	9

Source of data: Centre for Medicines Research (CMR) report CMR94-6R, The Strategy and Management of Successful Global R&D, August 1994 and CMR Poster presented at the Drug Information Association 30th Annual Meeting June 5–9, 1994, Washington, DC.

not known at the beginning, and an intelligent choice may only be made based on some structural similarity to drugs investigated earlier. Therefore, most initial studies are done with the standard species rat and dog. However, human kinetic and metabolism data should be collected as early as feasible in phase I to make the most appropriate species choices for longer term studies. The required duration of toxicological studies is determined by the intended treatment duration. For short treatment courses up to four weeks as with most antibiotics, three-month toxicological studies are sufficient for the clinical program and approval. Differences among the requirements for longer term clinical studies in different countries must be taken into account when coordinating the toxicological and clinical programs. The largest difference is in the requirement for Phase II trials of more than 4 weeks duration: US FDA guidelines require toxicological study durations identical to the intended human application, whereas EU and Japanese guidelines require 6- or even 12-month studies independent of treatment duration. This offers the possibility of an earlier phase II start in the U.S. It is good common practice to determine target organs and appropriate dose levels in shorter term or smaller pilot studies before embarking on the more costly long-term studies. However, the risk of missing the appropriate dose range can also be minimized by using more than the required minimum three doses in a study. A further option is to add additional animals to a longer term (e.g., 6-month) study and sacrifice some animals at half time to get an early indication that the study is on the right track. However, for ethical reasons, the toxicological program should be designed to avoid unnecessary repetition of studies with large numbers of animals. Generally, the most efficient toxicological program for a particular drug development should be planned by the toxicological expert with input by the whole project team rather than following a traditional standard pattern.

2. Phase I

Originally, the main objective of phase I studies was to establish the safety and tolerability of a new drug in healthy human volunteers. After starting with a single dose one to two orders of magnitude below the no effect dose in animals, this dose is increased in small steps with careful measurement and observation of a large number of laboratory and clinical parameters. Several such steps may be required until therapeutic drug levels are reached. After establishing single dose tolerability, this must be repeated in multi-dose studies whose treatment duration depends on the intended therapeutic dosing scheme. The total duration of this program depends greatly on the time required to evaluate a completed study sufficiently to justify initiating the next step. This can be done most efficiently if the whole sequence of studies is done in the same institution and by the same investigator, perhaps even within the company. Another consideration for the choice of study site may be the fact that phase I studies can be started in some European countries, such as Germany and U.K. approximately six months earlier than in the U.S. because extensive manufacturing and analytical reports on the formulation are not required in the data submission. In addition to safety information, many other valuable data are derived from phase I studies. Pharmacokinetic measurements give critical information on bioavailability and half life not infrequently very different from the animal data. This is important early guidance for formulation development. A low oral bioavailability of a costly drug substance may jeopardize the commercial success of a project unless a formulation with improved bioavailability can be developed. Low bioavailability also carries an increased risk of safety problems because of larger interindividual variations. If marketing considerations require a once daily dosing and a short half life makes this unlikely, the development of controlled release formulations should be started early. When possible, companies increasingly design their phase I programs to collect pharmacodynamic information, relevant to the intended therapeutic use, from healthy subjects. For example, bronchoprovocation or challenge studies give an important indication of the efficacy of asthma drugs. It may even be possible to determine the effective dose range with sufficient accuracy so that pivotal efficacy studies may be started immediately, parallel to formal dose finding studies, with considerable saving in total development time. Careful judgment by clinical experts is required in such decisions.

3. Clinical Development

Clinical development is the subject of a specific chapter in this book. Therefore, only a few general comments will be given. The duration of clinical studies determines most of the critical path for the largest part of the development program, and initially planned times for completing studies are often exceeded because estimated enrollment rates were too optimistic and countermeasures to prevent further delay were started too late. Important choices to be made, especially by companies doing parallel international development, are the country or continent for the study and whether to perform it through its own organization or contract it totally or in part to a Clinical Research Organization (CRO). In an international development effort, common understanding of goals and good coordination of activities between the regional departments are prerequisites for efficiency. Study sizes must be carefully calculated to offer the necessary statistical power for detecting the minimum therapeutic effect compatible with the approval criteria or a commercially viable product. In drug comparison studies, special attention must be given to the choice of the most suitable comparative drug. Different comparative drugs may be required in different regions or countries. Some of the most spectacular progress in reducing total drug development time has been made by shortening the time for trial data evaluation through continuous and/or remote entry of data during the study. In particular, this applies to interim analyses which may allow the next consecutive study to start earlier, when, for example, the effective dose range is sufficiently well established. The price for this faster study evaluation, however, is more work in the study planning and setup phase which, therefore, must be started early enough. The full benefit of a rapid study evaluation is obtained only when the next study is ready to start immediately. For this purpose, the design and preparations must also be as flexible as possible to allow for some last minute adjustments. For example, additional dose strengths of the formulation may be manufactured and stocked to avoid delays by a late change in the dosing scheme.

4. Manufacturing Development

Generally, clinical and toxicological studies are the most time consuming, and, typically, are the critical path activities of drug development. They also carry the highest risk of negative outcomes leading to project delay or even termination. However, drug substance and drug manufacturing issues are becoming increasingly complex and need careful attention in planning. Some reasons for this are more complex chemical structures—often stereoisomers—leading to larger number of synthesis steps and increased manufacturing cost, more frequent demand for controlled release or other special formulations, and more stringent regulatory requirements for GMP manufacturing. Newly developed technologies for advanced formulations often require lengthy optimization and scale-up, with considerable risk of unexpected problems and resulting delays. Every effort has to be made to use the final formulation in the large-scale, pivotal, phase III trials. Final formulation means that this formulation is supported by a sufficiently validated manufacturing scale process and sufficient stability data to minimize the need for further optimizations at the risk of changed properties. This rule is especially important for controlled release formulations because almost every formulation change requires a proof of bioequivalence with its inherent high risk of failure and the consequent repetition of clinical trials. For example, if development of the final formulation determines the initiation of phase III clinical development, the risk of study repetition must be carefully assessed against the later availability of decision-relevant data caused by waiting for the final formulation. An alternative decision would be to freeze the biokinetic specifications of the existing and not fully optimized formulation at the risk that further improvement of, e.g., stability, may not be feasible under this restriction. One of the positive developments in recent years was a trend to shorter regulatory approval times, especially in the U.S. When approval times took 2–4 years, most companies postponed production scale-up and commercial manufacturing preparations for this period. With current approval times of sometimes less than one year and the requirement to be ready for preapproval inspections within three months after submission, these activities must be done earlier, parallel to phase III studies, if launch delays after approval are to be avoided. Another reason for early acceptance of the final formulation is the need to complete stability studies in time to support approval and the intended shelf life at launch. Achievement of these tasks may also require earlier investments at a time when the efficacy and long term safety of the new drug are still under evaluation. The investment risk can be minimized if the company owns a multipurpose manufacturing plant capable of supplying the market for the first 2–3 years after launch.

The preceding paragraphs gave several examples demonstrating that starting new activities before the results of preceding studies are fully evaluated carries the increased risk that studies must be repeated because of inappropriate design. This risk must be carefully assessed against the chance of increased development speed. Alternative scenarios of outcomes and their consequences should be carefully considered. The final decision should be carried by broad consent. However, in many cases, it is advantageous to focus the plan on a go/no go decision and to reach this in the shortest possible time with the minimum amount of effort and data. In this way, many resources can be saved in the case of a negative outcome. In the event of a positive outcome, the missing studies can be started quickly without much loss in total time. The exact strategy selected will be specific to the project.

D. Stepwise Planning and Decision Points

Because of the uncertainties in drug development, effort would be wasted to plan the project from beginning to end in full detail. Even if the project finally belongs to the 10–15 percent of starts in preclinical development, which reach approval, the plan will most certainly be modified along the

Project Planning

way. It is sufficient to plan the work for the next phase or to the next decision point in full detail by defining each work package, its duration, prerequisites, and resource requirements, and the departments/persons responsible for its execution. For the following phases, an estimate of total time required should be made based on a listing of major, necessary studies, their sequence, and standard durations.

In addition to a company's standard decision points, additional decision points should be defined for recognized or probable critical issues so as not to waste resources on projects with limited chance of success. The project plan should aim to obtain the data for such decisions as early as possible even if the overall critical path analysis allows for investigations later. Examples are

potential for toxicity highlighted from chemical structure (e.g., phototoxicity or cancerogenicity),
feasibility of achieving the defined, unique, selling propositions,
feasibility of a commercially acceptable cost of goods,
feasibility of sufficient bioavailability for oral application,
feasibility of once daily application if required for marketing reasons, and
feasibility of a sufficiently stable formulation.

Some of these or other decision points may lead to a clear go/no go decision. Minimum performance requirements must be defined in advance. In other cases, several alternative courses of action may be possible depending on the outcome. Alternative scenario-type plans must be prepared to allow estimating the impact on total project time, commercial value, and resource requirements.

E. The Management of the Planning Process

Pharmaceutical development involves many disciplines and functions. Planning, therefore, is best done as a team effort with representatives from all the functions led by an experienced, independent, project manager. The functional representative's task is to define the methods, protocols, and study outlines required for the necessary proofs of efficacy, safety, and technical feasibility. Responsibility for making schedule commitments for the work packages and ensuring availability of needed resources is also part of the function. The project manager's task is to focus on the project target, overall time lines, and efficient use of resources so that nothing is overlooked and that the contributions of the different disciplines follow each other with the minimum amount of delay and with as much parallel work as feasible. One of the project manager's prime responsibilities is to ensure that every person involved in the project has the information necessary for contributing in the best and most timely manner.

The whole team should discuss every aspect of the plan in detail to address all possible effects of a particular experimental design or time plan in one area on the tasks under the responsibility of the other departments. Especially, regulatory consequences of, e.g., changes in study protocols or in formulation composition, must be carefully addressed to prevent later delays because of the need to repeat or add studies. This is of equal importance for plan adjustments reacting to technical or organizational problems which the executing department too often considers solely its own responsibility.

Furthermore, the team should not focus early on a single option for the whole or parts of the development plan but must outline several alternatives and consider their impact and consequences. To do this efficiently, team members must be open to proposals made by colleagues from other disciplines. For the same reason, the plan should not be kept secret but rather be openly available, e.g., in an electronic information system, to all stakeholders of the project.

For duration and completion planning of work packages, the project manager must, in principle, rely on the estimates given by the responsible team member. The project manager, however, should investigate the potential for time reduction especially if the activity is on the critical path and if the estimate is significantly longer than the duration given in the standard plan. In an optimized plan, it is normal that many work packages are very close to the critical path, i.e., their buffer times are only a few weeks or even days. Delayed start or small delays in their execution may quickly put them on the critical path. Therefore, it is essential that the project team and the project manager give the same attention to these activities as to the true critical path activities. Whenever possible, these activities should be started on the early start date, and any indications of threatening delay must be quickly communicated and acted on.

IV. PLANNING TOOLS AND SYSTEM SUPPORT

A. Network Plans

The concept of network plans was developed in parallel with general project management systems and is often wrongly taken as the essence of project management. Network plans are an extremely useful tool to organize most project activities so that the influence of time changes in each activity and the overall project completion time is clearly visible. The key output of a network plan is the critical path, that sequence of activities which determines the minimum duration of the project. It also defines lag times or buffers for all other activities. Reduction of the time to completion is possible only by doing critical path activities quicker or by rearranging the work to do activities in parallel instead of in sequence. Tracking of time must focus primarily on critical path activities (see Fig. 4).

B. The Standard Plan

Because pharmaceutical development of different drug candidates follows a broadly similar course largely set by scientific method and regulatory requirements, a formal "standard plan" is a very helpful tool. It summarizes the knowledge, experience, rules, and definitions of a development organization and serves as template and checklist for new project plans. Its main value is as assistance to ensure completeness of a specific project plan whereas the appropriate sequence of studies should be carefully optimized for each individual project using the considerations of the previous sections.

Standard plans are normally in the form of a network plan, showing

all activities (work packages) required to complete a project in terms of scientific, legal, and regulatory requirements
company internally defined decision points, milestones, evaluations, etc.
the linkage of these activities as derived from technical, scientific, ethical requirements or as internally defined
the standard time estimates for all work packages
the organizational unit responsible for the work package
the definition of the output of each work package

The computer network software calculates an overall duration and shows the critical path as well as time buffers. All activities in individual project plans should relate to these standard work packages through a description term or number.

To be a reliable tool, the standard plan must be regularly updated by the responsible project management department to include new regulatory and legal requirements and changed company procedures. Standard time estimates for experimental studies should reflect the time targets of the responsible departments for executing the task under normal conditions

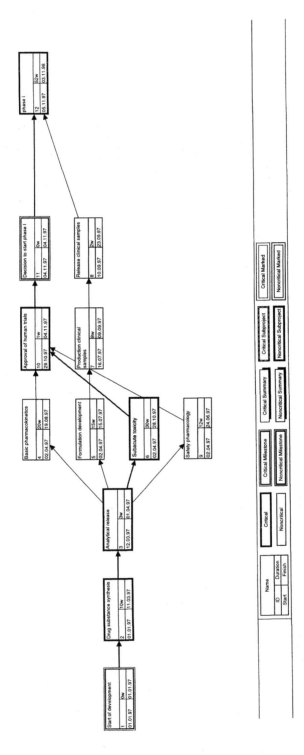

(A)

FIG. 4   Example of a small network plan in three data presentations: A. Network chart (PERT). B. Gantt chart showing critical and noncritical activities. C. Table showing calendar dates and buffer lengths (prepared using Microsoft Project®).

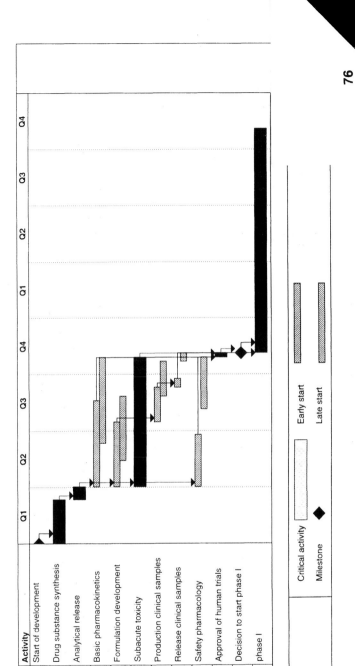

Number	Activity
1	Start of development
2	Drug substance synthesis
3	Analytical release
4	Basic pharmacokinetics
5	Formulation development
6	Subacute toxicity
7	Production clinical samples
8	Release clinical samples
9	Safety pharmacology
10	Approval of human trials
11	Decision to start phase I
12	phase I

Q1 Q2 Q3 Q4 Q1 Q2 Q3 Q4

Critical activity   Early start

Milestone ◆   Late start

(B)

Number	Activity	Duration	Start	Finish	Early start	Early finish	Late start	Late finish	Buffer
1	Start of development	0w	01.01.97	01.01.97	01.01.97	01.01.97	01.01.97	01.01.97	0w
2	Drug substance synthesis	10w	01.01.97	11.03.97	01.01.97	11.03.97	01.01.97	11.03.97	0w
3	Analytical release	3w	12.03.97	01.04.97	12.03.97	01.04.97	12.03.97	01.04.97	0w
4	Basic pharmacokinetics	20w	02.04.97	19.08.97	02.04.97	19.08.97	11.06.97	28.10.97	10w
5	Formulation development	15w	02.04.97	15.07.97	02.04.97	15.07.97	14.05.97	26.08.97	6w
6	Subacute toxicity	30w	02.04.97	28.10.97	02.04.97	28.10.97	02.04.97	28.10.97	0w
7	Production clinical samples	8w	16.07.97	09.09.97	16.07.97	09.09.97	27.08.97	21.10.97	6w
8	Release clinical samples	2w	10.09.97	23.09.97	10.09.97	23.09.97	22.10.97	04.11.97	6w
9	Safety pharmacology	12w	02.04.97	24.06.97	02.04.97	24.06.97	06.08.97	28.10.97	18w
10	Approval of human trials	1w	29.10.97	04.11.97	29.10.97	04.11.97	29.10.97	04.11.97	0w
11	Decision to start phase I	0w	04.11.97	04.11.97	04.11.97	04.11.97	04.11.97	04.11.97	0w
12	phase I	52w	05.11.97	03.11.98	05.11.97	03.11.98	05.11.97	03.11.98	0w

FIG. 4 Continued

(C)

without abnormal resource constraints and unexpected problems. When available, benchmarking data from high performing competitors should be used to set the standard durations.

Network plans and standard plans are not very suitable for representing repetitive tasks, such as production and release of drug substance or formulation supply in numerous consecutive batches. These important activities should be tracked separately in suitable task lists or action plans. A similar situation applies to certain actions required mostly in preparing and optimizing the plan, such as collecting information and opinions.

C. Information Systems

1. Requirements for Single Project Planning

When starting on a new project plan, the team lists tasks, defines work packages, determines predecessor/successor sequences and asks for time duration estimates. The clearest way to present and discuss this information is the classical bar or Gantt chart. Initially, this is probably drawn on a flip chart but, as soon as the information starts consolidating, it is useful to document and organize it by using one of the many available project management softwares. This allows quick and easy changes, presentations in various levels of detail or in various time-frames, "what-if" tests of alternative ways to proceed, and, generally, a very nice and clear presentation of the data.

However, the benefit of using network software for project optimization seems limited. The critical path of a project, typically, is evident without computer help, and the effect of possible measures for time reduction may be evaluated easily on paper. However, it is useful to see the early and late start dates of noncritical activities and to use this information for resource scheduling. Many software packages allow entering original and revised plan dates for convenient tracking and preparation of progress reports.

For these reasons, the author recommends the use of networking software for pharmaceutical development projects. The systems may be PC-based or mainframe. Usually, PC-based software can also be run on client/server networks using a variety of operating systems. Many of them can also exchange their data with common data banks, e.g., ORACLE. Some of the more frequently used systems are listed in Table 7. Detailed information on the functionality and system requirements of the different products can easily be obtained from vendors, e.g., through their Internet presentations. Reviews and comparisons can also be found in a variety of computer publications, e.g., in [3]. The choice of a system also depends on the ap-

TABLE 7

Project Scheduling and Network Plan Software

Product	Vendor
Multiuser systems:	
ARTEMIS 7000, 9000, Prestige	CSC Artemis
Open Plan	Welcom Software
Project Planner (P3)	Primavera
P/X	Project Software & Dev., Inc. (PSDI)
Single project systems:	
Fast Track Schedule	AEC Software
Micro Planner X-Pert	Micro Planning Intl
Microsoft Project	Microsoft
Project Scheduler 7	Scitor Corp.
Superproject	Computer Associates
Suretrack Project Manager	Primavera
Texim Project	Welcom Software
Time Line	Timeline Solutions

proach to documenting multiproject information, as discussed below. A few programs allow simultaneous access by several users in a network and can cover the needs of single and multiproject planning in the same system. More and more of the single user systems simulate this capability by connecting to an external data base using ODBC (open data base connectivity) or SQL (Structured query language).

Because all activities of a project may not be well represented in a network plan, the project manager needs additional software tools to list and track those. Standard data base or spreadsheet software is usually suitable. Modern software solutions integrate data bases, network systems and communication tools into one user-friendly surface. A recent example is PAVONE GroupProject based on Lotus Notes. However, specific recommendations would be soon antiquated because of the rapid development of new software.

2. Multiproject Planning Systems

The different functional departments in an organization need an overview of their ongoing and planned activities to track and schedule resources.

Relational data bases are usually sufficient for this purpose, and networking capability is not essential.

The system requirements for multiproject management within departments are very different depending on the amount and complexity of data and the number and geographical distribution of data entry points. Therefore, it does not seem feasible or even desirable to cover the needs of all development departments with a single system. However, access to the data should be provided to project managers and others needing them for their work with a similar user-friendly surface.

3. Management Information Systems

Management needs information on project plans, status, and progress at an upper, condensed level. Typically, this is the level of milestones, general and specifically defined decision points, and time-critical activities. Such data should be kept in a data base easily accessible to all members of a defined group of managers.

4. System Integration

The three-level project planning and tracking system described above represents the reality in many pharmaceutical companies today. Obviously identical work packages are documented redundantly in separate systems with the need to duplicate and harmonize data entry. This may seem odd in today's age of advanced data processing. Ideally all of the tasks described above would be handled by a single system requiring the entry of each event only once. The reality, however, has shown that such integrated systems would make too many compromises on user requirements or be extremely difficult to handle. Many such projects have been unsuccessful because they could only partially replace parallel data banks with the same data. Today the trend is to compatibility of data banks allowing different applications to work with their data. In such a system, plan and actual dates of work packages would be downloaded from the departmental multiproject systems into the project manager's network system, and milestones and decision points uploaded into the management information system. Ideally, the system would provide the project manager with comparison lists for the data from the different sources with the possibility to mark the intended up- and down-loads. Such a system would reflect the reality of a large working organization, where differences in information and planning will not be avoided. They would, however, be rapidly detected and acted upon. It is hoped that rapid software development will make such solutions possible in the near future. New developments known as Intranet or Data warehouse point in this direction.

SUGGESTED FURTHER READING

1. M Mathieu. *New Drug Development: A Regulatory Overview*. Cambridge, MA: Parexel International Corporation, 1990.
2. Section III: Medicine Discovery and Development in Bert Spilker, *Multinational Pharmaceutical Companies. Principles and Practices*, 2nd ed. New York: Raven Press, 1994.
3. N H King, *Project Management: On Time and On Budget*. PC Magazine, April 11, 1995, p 165.

4

Perspectives from Other Industries: Best Practice and Evolving Trends

Ian Reynolds

Logica UK Limited
London, England

I. INTRODUCTION

In peacetime, the defense industry was once thought to be slow to achieve, muddled and yet profitable with the constant changes to specification and costs being picked up by the taxpayer. The changing defense procurement scenario in the late 80s required a drastic change in the methods and the culture within the industry. This section of the book is concerned with the developments in the management approach to a particular large project that was transformed from certain disaster into a resounding success.

In the defense industry, production runs are generally low volume and design and development is a one product exercise. Accordingly, the whole business is run on a project basis covering all aspects from cradle to grave of a particular weapon system except for the weapon use. Although other industries may be similar to this model, the majority are not because projects are concerned only with the initial development and production and/or operational use is in another branch of the company. Perhaps, another difference is that the customer has a very large organization, traditionally with access to all levels of the company and accounts. Furthermore, the customer is purchasing the equipment on behalf of the service user (who are very powerful and influential in their own right when it comes to procurement decisions).

In summary, the project manager has a vast number of the customer's staff to satisfy while making sure that the eventual equipment user is satisfied. In this respect, the defense project manager is a combination of a program manager and a project manager.

II. PROGRAM MANAGEMENT VS. PROJECT MANAGEMENT

The simple differences between a program manager and a project manager are that

a program manager manages the benefits accruing from the use of the project deliverables from inception to realization of the benefits through operational use of the deliverables;

whereas the project manager aims to achieve the deliverables on time at the right technical and quality standard and at minimum cost, there is no concern with the use that the deliverables will be put to achieve the users' benefits.

It is beyond the scope of this section to deal with the elements of program management in the role of a defense project manager, so, the following sections concentrate on the project management role.

III. PROJECT MANAGEMENT

It is important to understand the role of the project manager within the defense industry and how it relates to the functional organization. The company in question was organized into different directorates. These were Operations (fabrication, assembly and test), Engineering [i.e., Electronic design, Mechanical design, Test (not production equipment), Production engineering], Commercial, Procurement, Projects, Product Support, Business Development, Quality, and Personnel.

Before the major changes (detailed below), the role of the project manager varied from being a liaison between "engineering" and the customer to being in total charge of the business. The major change gave the project manager the responsibility to:

- delegate authority from and answerable to the company managing director
- direct the work of all other functions on project business
- decide project policy, strategy, methods of reporting and managing
- authorize all expenditure and changes to the program to maximize the business
- hold the project contingency and to manage the profit and loss account
- be the prime business and customer focus
- manage the project business to achieve the deliverables on time, on budget, and to the correct technical and quality standards
- manage the project business to ensure short-term cash flow, medium-term profitability, and long-term business growth.

The functional directorates were in charge of the staff who were not project specific and they were more concerned (eventually) with how to do it rather than what to do. The project manager was the person who delegated what to do and when.

IV. CONTROL OF PROJECTS

A. Background and Situation Status

The need for the major change was created by a change in Defense procurement policy from "cost plus" (where any time spent on the project was chargeable to the customer with profit added—consequently delays and problems were more profitable than achieving on time!) to "fixed price" (where the industry took the risk).

This change came at a time of a shrinking marketplace with serious overcapacity in Europe and the U.S.A. The increased competition with the new penalties of fixed price and liquidated damages started to focus the industry toward changing to survive. Internally, the new fixed-price contracts were consistently late with payments delayed and reduced profitability. Our reputation was being seriously damaged, and there was too much firefighting by the senior managers.

The opportunity to change came when different divisions were combined as part of the industry rationalization with the project managers using vastly different systems to control the business. To compound this problem, the various functional heads within the organization, who controlled the staff, also tried to control the project progress without the responsibility for achievement. As they were only really concerned with ensuring that their own staff was successful, the projects reeled from one "functional baron's" whims to the next. This was great in the cost-plus days but not when we had to make a profit on fixed price contracts.

B. Knowing What to Aim For

The projects were assessed to see which problem areas really existed. It soon became clear that there was little or no control and that the major problem areas were

- no ability to measure spending vs. achievement or cost to completion
- No mechanisms to use the program to
  - control the schedule
  - predict schedule problems (rather than when they are fait accompli)
  - replan when changes occur
- no processes to ensure that only one person is accountable for spending and achievement, to give all staff access to the program, or to create a team spirit that looks upon achievement as the norm rather than the exception.

This gave rise to a number of primary issues that had to be resolved if we were to remain in business. In summary they were

- to break the work into manageable packages
- to give accountability, responsibility, and authority to members of a project team reporting to the project manager
- to have a resourced "PERT" network with each package of work linked together
- to have good communication of changing program priorities
- to report variances to plan and the appropriate actions to recover
- to ensure that all staff had clear roles and responsibilities

- to ensure that a continuous improvement mentality was introduced into all processes.

C. Management of Change

The business was divided into 23 projects. The largest one completely dwarfed the rest. This project was in serious need of changes because of costs overrunning, no forecast of the future costs, and a three year history of thirteen major changes agreed to by the customer because of industry nonperformance. Although the project was large (spending about £10 million a week at the peak and the largest U.K. Defence Land System procurement), cost controls had totally broken down with an average of 66 work packages for every engineer! The revenue stream from the customer was still continuing, albeit there was very serious worry that the project would soon collapse.

A team of thirty staff, from all levels, was colocated in an open plan office with an aim to develop a new system of operation and to implement it without any delay to the revenue stream. Although we knew what to do, the "functional barons" could have been our downfall because the staff followed them so closely. The key to success was to develop and implement two initiatives, one to control projects and one to control and improve the functional technical excellence of the company processes. The basic game plan was to get the "barons" involved with the team, set them hard targets for achieving technical excellence to keep them busy, and then, to implement changes in the project organization which would remove their powers.

The project changes were introduced. Then the "barons" were reintroduced, after about six months, to supporting the projects rather than controlling them. This gave the new project organization time to settle down, and everyone knew who their boss was for project achievement.

The changeover was handled with extreme care so that the actual workers (rather than the managers) did not stop their work, but it was now controlled in a different way. The project staff attitudes were grouped in being willing to change with no effort, change with persuasion, or would not change categories. Some of the latter category were so against change that they had to be released. Although the staff was persuaded with buy-in to the development of the process, the actual implementation was by substituting the project manager, followed by team building and a strict program of activities that stretched the staff, so that they had no time to question the changes. Artificial crises were instigated to give tough but achievable targets when there was any sign that the staff was moving away from implementation.

When the new system was in place, the staff was consulted within preprogrammed continuous improvement meetings, so that their builds could be incorporated within the basic framework. This was a tough time when the whole process could have collapsed. Thorough preparation was necessary. The most significant factor was removal of the "functional barons" to concentrate on their functional excellence.

A number of barriers were faced which had to be overcome, such as

- fear of failure and having the confidence to win
- resistance to change
- lack of understanding of the new roles and responsibilities and how to act as a team

These are predominant people issues so, a dedicated Personnel representative was added to the project management team to facilitate progress in this area. The areas of change affected the whole company, particularly the areas of Project Management, Operations, Engineering, Quality, and Procurement.

D. Critical Success Factors

The critical success factors associated with the change were

- giving the "barons" something else to do while the project processes were implemented
- getting control of the work, costs, and future forecasts
- keeping the revenue stream going, almost irrespective of short-term achievement.

The first two were achieved by implementing technical excellence and the project management framework changes detailed below. The last required a significant investment in presentations and openness with the customer about the new processes. The customer's project manager was invited to a number of brainstorming sessions during the development of the processes. Although he had observer status, he quickly became involved with the change and was given actions like everyone else. When it came to the actual change, he was already part of the process, and he has given lots of support to help his colleagues and staff make the leap of faith to a new process.

E. The Work Breakdown Structure

Different types of work breakdown structure were examined including combinations of deliverable at the top level and functional at the lower levels.

The major problem with any type of functional package of work is the high cost of coordination when changes occur and the possibility that functional empires will be rebuilt. Accordingly, a deliverable-based work breakdown structure was adopted which had a repeating framework until a single manager could effectively manage the work. This meant that the smallest packages had to have a real manager (rather than an engineer who was not interested in costs or achievement) and was multifunctional involving staff from different departments and skill sets. The generic work breakdown structure is shown in Fig. 1.

The basic concept for development (for example) is that the work is broken down into a number of subsystems and overall test equipment according to the output of the system design area. This also defines the integration requirements and interfaces between subsystems. The system test area is responsible for the certification against the requirements. Each subsystem is further broken down into sub-subsystems with their system design and integration, subsystem test equipment, and test areas. Each level has its own management, so that it is a self contained entity that could easily be let to a subcontractor or undertaken in-house. The smallest package of work was aptly named a task package that had a resourced network, a budget, and a set of requirements passed down from above in the work breakdown structure. All the networks were linked together to produce an overall program for the project. The structure does not have a separate package for "Quality" as it was incumbent on the whole staff to build quality into the product and not to have someone else responsible for their quality.

The benefits from this type of structure are that

- it ensures that all areas are covered including subcontractors;
- it links deliverables into the contract and identifies each deliverable cost;
- historical data is independent of organizational change;
- it is not parochial in terms of department, function, or directorate, and it encourages interfunctional teamwork;
- it gives clear accountability and responsibility to managers;
- design reviews are easier as each level is the design authority;
- it is flexible with project size;
- the structure can increase bidding efficiency.

Each of the other areas (Production and In service) had a similar work breakdown structure so that there was a clear relationship between development and production of the same deliverable at each level.

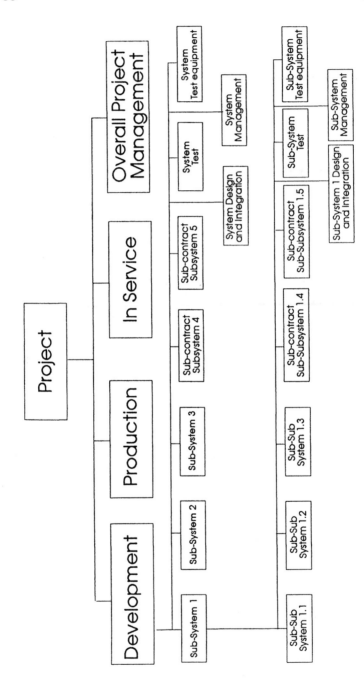

FIG. 1   The generic work breakdown structure showing the repeating breakdown.

F. The Organizational Structure

The key to efficiency in running a project is to provide a framework in which everyone can work effectively. Although the work breakdown structure is this basic framework, the successful completion of the project must be facilitated by an organization structure that ensures clear roles, responsibilities, and accountability without over- or underlap. The actual organization put in place to achieve this consisted of a core team of managers and a project team of managers and workers. The organization structure was, essentially, a population of the work breakdown structure with a few exceptions within the core team.

1. The Core Team

The core team consisted of a colocated (as much as was practical) team of top managers down to subsystem level. Each member of the core team had a one-to-one relationship with members of the customer's and user's organizations. The simplified organization structure is shown in Fig. 2.

Each member was supplied and functionally owned by the directorate/function/department with the necessary skills to undertake the job. For example, the Chief Engineer was from the Engineering Directorate, the Program Coordinator from the Project Management Directorate, a subcontract Task Group Manager (TGM) from the Procurement Directorate and other TGMs from Engineering. This was a fundamental element of the whole structure and project control, and the boss did not need to know how to undertake his subordinate's job. The boss' job was to coordinate and manage the various disciplines to achieve his deliverable, i.e., what and when to do it and not how.

This multifunctional team was administered for the duration of the project by the Project Manager as a department undertaking the short-term "feeding and watering." The long-term career of the staff and its technical ability to undertake the job was looked after by the directorate/function that owned them.

Communication across different project phases (all of which happen at the same time in mid-project) was at multiple levels as each Development TGM had a corresponding Production Group manager both of whom were responsible for the same deliverable.

The areas outside the work breakdown structure population were

- the project Control Manager and staff
- the Boards of Directors (BODs).

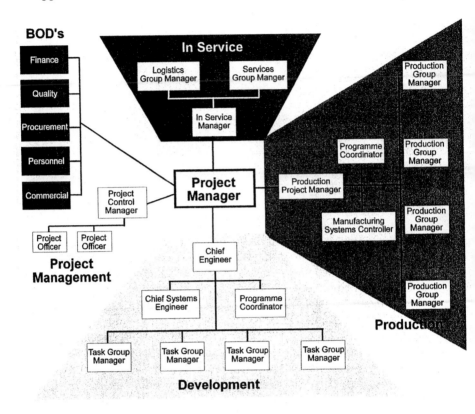

FIG. 2   The simplified core team organizational structure.

The Project Control Managers responsibility was to facilitate achievement across the three project phases and to formulate options and recommendations for improvement and variance resolution. An example of this was the missile boxes. When the Production Project Manager tried to deliver the first tranche of missiles, the user rejected them, even though the customer had agreed and signed off on the design. The In Service Manager could not persuade the user to accept them because the design of the boxes was impractical for use in his scenario. The Production staff wanted to keep producing the old design but the Chief Engineer was happy to stop production for six months while he developed an alternative design. As Project Manager, I wanted the revenue stream to continue through deliveries. The Project Control Manager persuaded the user to accept the current design while a new design was developed which would be retrofitted to the first batch at a later date by the In Service team. Accordingly, each project phase was coordinated to achieve the requirements of the Project Manager.

The BODs were the advisors to the project. Their role was to feed any Directorate potential changes into the project, to feedback the project requirements to the functional directorates, and to support the project's progress. An example of this was the Procurement BOD who was tasked to examine the top 10 issues on each of the subcontractors. Instead of resolving these individually, he was asked to look laterally across the issues to determine if a change in company or project procurement policy would improve the subcontractor's performance. In this example, there were 21 key issues across 17 major subcontractors, seventeen of which were directly within the control of the company to improve. The Procurement BOD, then, was required to formulate an improvement program for his directorate's technical excellence.

2. The Project Team

Outside the core team were the first line managers—Task Package Coordinators (TPCs) and their staffs. These TPCs were the first reports to the Task Group Managers (or equivalent) and commanded a team of eight to ten staff mostly from the TPC's department but not exclusively. This multifunctional team was responsible for creating the deliverable in the lowest level in the work breakdown structure. Both of these TPCs and their staffs were located within their directorate/functional/departmental structure. Accordingly the TPCs had two bosses:

1. for the project work (The Task Group Manager), who said what to do and when to complete it
2. for functional excellence (The Departmental Head), who told him how to do it.

It was very important to ensure that the two bosses did not both require reporting for the same thing. Because the functional barons were used to trying to do both of these roles (and failing), it was necessary to break their power during the change, and hence, the functional excellence initiative was implemented at the same time. Figure 3 illustrates the relationship between the directorates/functions/departments and the core team.

The TPC evaluated the probability of undertaking current and future tasks within the budget, timescales, and to the correct technical/quality standards. Should the probability be below 90%, then, the TPC would bring this potential problem to his departmental head for guidance while warning the TGM. The departmental head may raise this problem to the functional

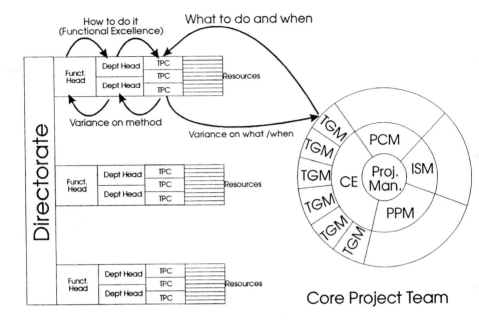

Core Project Team

Functional Organization

FIG. 3   The Matrix Organization: The relationship between the Functional Teams and the Project Team in a matrix structure with supporting responsibilities.

head for guidance if he could not solve the problem. Should this avenue of functional excellence fail, then, it became likely that nothing could be done to achieve the task without a change in the budget, timescales, or technical standard (quality was never compromised). The TPC would, then bring a program variance to his TGM for resolution. The variance would also be raised to the function for continuous improvement of functional excellence through real examples of where the original functional guidance on "how to do it" had failed to be achieved. In this way, the TPC has the benefit of excellent functional support without the conflicts that a single "boss" would bring.

G. Framework of Control

1. The Reporting and Authority Levels

When a variance is raised to the TGM, he will attempt to resolve the issue through an optimization of his task groups. As he is the Design Authority

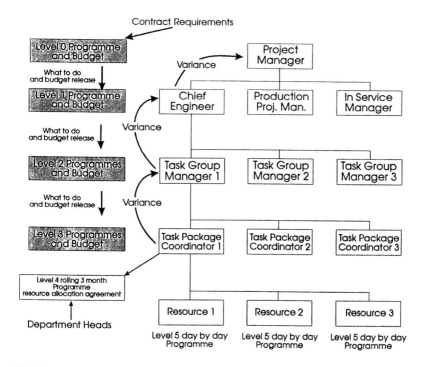

FIG. 4 The program breakdown: Program requirements are passed down and any variances to program achievement are brought to the level where they can be resolved and no further.

for his deliverable, he has the authority to change the technical compliance and timescales as long as it does not affect the next level up program (see Fig. 4). Should the TGM be unable to resolve the issue, then the TGM brings the variance to the Chief Engineer who would try to resolve it through a reoptimization of his program phase. Again, should this not be possible he will bring it to the Project Manager who will attempt to resolve it within the terms and conditions of the contract. In this way, problems are only brought to the level at which they can be resolved rather than raising all problems directly to upper management who would spend all their time firefighting.

If the problem could be resolved through release of contingency, then, the coordinator/manager at any level has the option to raise a business case to facilitate release of contingency (held by the Project Manager). This business case must indicate that a release of contingency is the most cost-

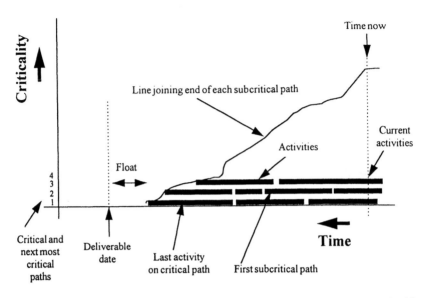

FIG. 5   The criticality measure: Each activity path had its own measure of criticality dependent on the float to the deliverable data.

effective avenue for the project. Figure 4 shows how the requirements and budget were passed down and variances to plan flowed up for resolution.

Each level creates a plan that is integrated at the next level. Computerized plans are produced for levels 0 to 3. The level 4 plan is a rolling quarter-year plan created against which individual staff were assigned with agreement between the department heads and the TPC. The level 5 plan is a day-by-day individual plan created for a week and agreed on between the TPC and his staff.

Each area had a degree of management flexibility, before variances were brought to higher levels for resolution, that depended on how critical the activity was to the deliverables and milestones. (The next section indicates how the criticality of activities was measured.) The computerized network plans were updated weekly in line with a strictly followed timetable, as shown in the following sections.

2. Key Performance Indicators

To ensure that the project was continuing and improving, a number of Key Performance Indicators (KPIs) were developed. These were aimed at showing whether the changes and the project progress were to plan. Specialist

KPIs, which depended upon program deliverables, were developed for the key areas, and more general ones of efficiency and program criticality were used across the project. Monitoring actual costs against planned costs is of little use unless the achievement is also measured. The efficiency KPI used was

$$\text{Efficiency} = \frac{\text{actual cost} / \text{planned cost}}{\text{actual achivement} / \text{planned achievement}}$$

The criticality KPI was particularly useful because the project was large with multiple critical and subcritical paths to each major deliverable/milestone. A backward pass was calculated from the overall network and each subcritical path noted with its float. A graph shown in Fig. 5 was drawn with each critical/subcritical path showing the end date. This shows how the criticality of the activities was related to the deliverable date. Accordingly, management action could be prioritized by the degree of float appropriate to each activity with a problem. In this way, management time could be optimized by concentrating on those problems critical to the deliverable success, and the staff members knew where their tasks fitted into the overall plan and how critical their contributions were.

The criticality KPI represented a trend showing whether or not the program criticality was improving. An arbitrary date was chosen before the deliverable date (shown in Fig. 6 as 5 weeks).

Then, the area under the graph was calculated and plotted as the Criticality KPI every week, as shown in Fig. 7.

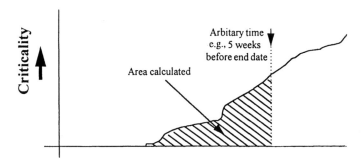

FIG. 6 The area of criticality: This area is a measure of how critical the program is.

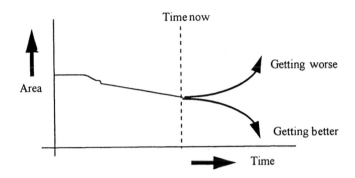

FIG. 7   The Criticality KPI: The weekly trend showing whether the program was improving or getting worse.

As the area increased, the program was becoming more critical and, hence, more unlikely to be achieved, and, as the area reduced, the program was becoming easier to achieve.

3. The Variances and How to Control Them

Variances to the program (or costs) were raised by any level within the organization. A strict timetable of meetings and variance resolution was followed to ensure that variances were handled quickly. (Previously, problems were hidden through fear of failure, so that, when they eventually surfaced, they were usually irreparable.) The message was that failure was not a failure to achieve the program, so revealing a failure in good time eventually became part of the new culture. Accordingly, there was a great deal more openness in the organization with problems discussed rather than hidden. This timetable is shown in Fig. 8.

Armed with variances and criticality information, the best use of management time could be achieved by accepting noncritical variances and resolving those with a severe impact on the deliverables. Compression of timescales was also achieved using the "backward path" information because saving weeks off the critical path without looking at the next most subcritical path was pointless. The Project Managers weekly meeting evaluated the elements in Fig. 9 that formed the agenda for the meeting.

The risk register also was a fundamental element of the program for estimating future costs, variances, and the actions of special action teams.

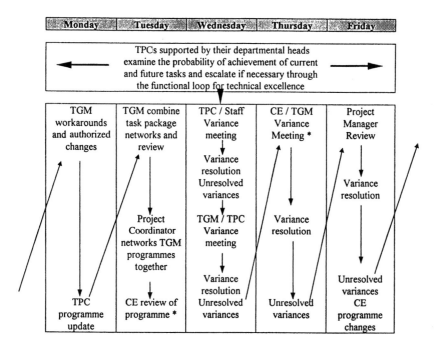

FIG. 8 The weekly variance resolution cycle: The program was updated every week with fixed times for all variance meetings and resolution.

4. Special Action Teams

Special action teams were set up to undertake off-line activities, such as

- cycle compression,
- risk mitigation to reduce or alleviate the effect of future risks,
- contract amendment bids (these ranged from £20 thousand to £84 million), and
- process enhancements.

It was essential to keep these activities off-line, otherwise, the teams charged with achieving the program would have been diverted, and conflicts of priorities would have produced an overall delay.

Progress	Costs	Variances	Risks	KPI's
• Consistent with last week's expectations Future programme undertaken in same time Equipment defects • Review of special action teams progress	• In line with programme • Costs left to go within cost to completion budget • Review of savings opportunities	• Number raised • Number solved • Number with plan to solve • Number without resolution - help required • Criticality	• Review of risk register - probability of future risks being realized • Review of new realized risks • Review of risk aversion strategies • Review of special action teams progress	• Review of all KPI's appropriate to Project Manager
Review in more depth during meeting if answers not on programme/costs or as expected. Particularly critical variances.				

FIG. 9   The Project Manager's weekly meeting topics: Every element of the program was reviewed weekly to ensure that the correct progress was being made.

H. The Outcome

The changes introduced had a major impact on the company organization and on the structures reporting, internally and externally, to subcontractors and the customer. The path to success was difficult, and many staff members could not cope with the changes, in particular, where first level managers were promoted to be TGMs in the initial change. Some of these new TGMs had difficulty cutting the link between with the actual workers and could not cope with reliance on management information as they were now managers of managers rather than managers of doers.

Initially, the customer was skeptical because of great influence in the project direction without the burden of responsibility. The customer also thought that the accounting side might be a potential problem because postcontract audits, in the past, had been able to delve into the cost of individual items, such as ball point pens! This was not the sort of detail that was necessary to manage the project, and the changes created larger packages of work that could not be so easily assessed. Although it was difficult to persuade the customer that the new methodology was going to create a success without its direct involvement in industrial decisions, when successful results started to become obvious, the customer became very enthusiastic. The success increased throughout the project (which lasted six years

Parameter		Before the changes	After the changes
Organization	Structure and relationship with Customer	Functional. Project Management acted as liaison between the customer and Engineering. Relationship between Customer and Production, Quality and Commercial, ad hoc with no coordination.	Multifunctional. Matched to the Work Breakdown Structure with all interfaces to the Customer co-ordinated by the core team. Published customer pairing arrangements covering all functions based upon deliverables
	Relationship with the sub-contractors	Multifunctional uncoordinated approach. Contract, workstatement and programme not linked together.	Single interface for deliverable Part of Work Breakdown Structure and programme
	Staffing	Split up by functions in different buildings. Accountable to the functions (not the project) and skills appropriate to a single function.	Core Team Co-located. All staff accountable to the project for their deliverable achievement and to their function for their professional ability. Multifunctional training introduced. Continuous improvement methodologies ingrained into all processes.
	Attitude	'Don't ask me, it's not mine and even if it was mine it would not be my fault'	'Can do/Will do/Have done'
	Culture	• The more we waste the larger our profits (cost plus) • I expect someone else will tell me if I have done something wrong (it's easier than checking it oneself) • I don't care where the work comes from or goes to. As long as I do my bit I won't get criticized	• Problems don't exist - only opportunities • I am responsible, this is what I am doing and by when. • I know why I am doing this and how it fits into the overall business. • When it's complete, I will autograph it as I am proud of it.

FIG. 10   The results of the change.

after the major changes) and the customer wanted the methodology to become the industry standard. Through the subcontractors to the project, the basic principles have been incorporated into a number of different companies within the industry. The major achievements that were created (apart from a successful conclusion to the project) are given in Fig. 10.

These changes allowed the program to be successfully completed. At the formal end of development, the customer commented:

Parameter		Before the changes	After the changes
Programme	Ownership	'Project Management' with no buy-in from any other function.	Ownership was an integral part of the new philosophy and everyone owned the programme for the task or package that they were responsible for.
	Bad interfaces (illogical links)	500 was termed good!	Zero was achieved and maintained. This created no surprises.
	Resources	Not linked to cost structure (Work Breakdown Structure) or the programme.	Integral part of the Work Breakdown structure. Each activity was resourced by skill, skill level, quantity and costs.
Cost	Charging numbers	53,000 - equates to 66 for every engineer! This was totally out of control and not linked to the programme.	Approx. 300 with owners and programmes all integrated into the Work Breakdown Structure and programme.
	Cost to Complete	Unknown. Project Management guess based upon scant knowledge of future programme.	Fully integrated into costing system.
Risk		Assessment of risks undertaken by Engineering but no link to costs or programme. No risk mitigation plans, accountability or evaluation of contingency requirements.	Fully integrated risk assessment. management and avoidance/recovery systems with positive spend to save attitude at all levels in the organisation.

FIG. 10   Continued

The product will be a highly effective system that meets its design requirements and, in some areas, in excess of specification. This reflects great credit primarily on U.K. industry.

Such success has seldom, if ever, been achieved for such a complicated and sophisticated weapon system anywhere in the world.

5

Managing an International Project Team

Donald N. Cooper

Hoffmann-La Roche
Nutley, New Jersey

I. OVERVIEW

A great deal of expertise and experience is needed to effectively manage an international project team. The ideal project leader must possess a multitude of skills and motivate other professional managers productively in a multicultural and multidisciplinary matrix environment. This individual must provide a global and balanced perspective to the organization while evaluating critical issues and must fully appreciate and understand the regulatory and business requirements of key markets around the world. In addition, the project leader must think strategically, have the interest and patience to delve into project details, often in areas in which he is not expert, have an extensive background in drug development, and have a working knowledge of and appreciation for project management and financial tools and techniques.

For any one individual to become knowledgeable and equally proficient in such a wide range of skills would certainly be a remarkable achievement. However, there are a few critical personal traits and project experiences which, honed properly, provide the leader with sufficient tools to manage a team successfully. Clearly, unambiguous support from senior management is a prerequisite, for without it, less than desirable outcomes usually result. The proven ability to communicate effectively and the consistent demonstration of successful achievement, drive, commitment, and enthusiasm are key drivers for success. The project leader must pay a great deal of attention to organizing his team with particular emphasis on enumerating and agreeing on individual and team expectations, responsibilities, and scope of authority. By building on this foundation and by ensuring that team operating procedures are in place and are supported by the organization, the project leader and the project leader's team will be well equipped to face challenges.

II. ORGANIZATIONAL SUPPORT AND COMMITMENT TO PROJECT TEAMS AND PROJECT MANAGEMENT

To effectively manage an international team, a project leader must overcome national, functional, and organizational boundaries which pose obstacles to the achievement of the stated mission. To be successful, it is paramount that senior management provide clear support and consistently articulate their expectations that all members of their organization be aligned with the goals and efforts of the project team.

A successful project leader must be able to effectively and efficiently address complex project-related issues and problems which invariably come up during drug development. Paramount among these is the importance placed on building an international team from a group of individuals, who come from fairly diverse disciplines, backgrounds, and cultures, and demonstrating the capability to consistently and successfully overcome organizational roadblocks which negatively affect the project team's performance. A project leader must count on the assistance of senior management when needed and be assured that their support is communicated wholeheartedly to the organization as unambiguously as possible. This support must be consistently reinforced at key times throughout the long drug development process.

Supporting the role of the project leader and providing this individual with the tools necessary to be successful means that management also has a significant responsibility to assure that their message comes across loud and clear to everyone in their organization, and, in particular, to those individuals in positions to significantly affect and/or be influenced by the project leader's and the international project team's performance. Management must articulate the "boundaries" within which they expect the team to operate, the importance they place in the project leader's role, and the level of commitment and support they expect this individual to receive from all members of the organization. Because of the length of time required to develop a new chemical entity, the repetitiveness of these important messages becomes critical, particularly because it is often observed that over time some key individuals selectively remember only what is expected of them. Lack of visible support by senior management poses significant difficulties for the project leader and affects the leader's ability to manage the team effectively.

What level of responsibility and authority can a project leader expect to receive from management? Depending on the organization, that would depend upon how the project leader's role is perceived and the degree of empowerment which is really provided. The authority inherent in the job does not evolve primarily from a job description, but builds over time from the decisions, processes, and management behavior evident everyday in the organization. The project leader is, however, the one individual within the organization empowered with the basic responsibility of providing the overall direction and coordination for a project through all the development phases to complete it on schedule and within budget while maximizing the commercial potential of the company's assets. As such, this individual plays a key role in helping the organization achieve its overall corporate objectives.

Because the project leader's primary task is optimally integrating the efforts of all international team members who are contributing to the project, it is critical that management ensure that the role of project leader is considered a fairly senior level position in the organization. This becomes particularly important in a team environment where it is difficult for someone who is perceived as a junior in an organization to effectively manage other high level executives. In a matrix organization, if the project leader's organizational stature is not at least equivalent to that of the most senior member of the team and/or the project leader does not possess the political and organizational clout necessary to effectively influence and lead others, despite the stated position, the project leader will find it quite difficult to fulfill the leadership role and will wind up primarily doing the job expected of a project coordinator, not a leader.

Where, and to whom in an organization the project leader reports depends on a multitude of organizational factors, i.e., the size of the company and the company's bureaucracy, the number of projects which need to be managed on an international scale, the scope of the projects, the expectations the organization has for the role of the project leader, the appropriate level of senior executive who the organization feels is needed to resolve key organizational and project-related roadblocks, etc. Care must be taken to ensure that the reporting relationship is sufficiently high up in the organization to provide project leaders with the "clout" they need to get the job done, yet not so high that they lose touch with everyday reality.

A. Communication

A project leader needs to interact with senior executives on a fairly frequent basis. It is important for the project leader to build strong relationships with key organizational players who can "make things happen" and over time to pay particular attention to ensure that these executives develop the confidence in the project leader's leadership and management ability. Given the significant project issues which need to be addressed on a daily basis and the extensive time commitment usually demanded of any individual working within a project team environment, it is fairly easy to minimize the importance of networking as a "nice to do" activity. However, this would be a major mistake and could certainly come back to haunt the project leader in the future, particularly if the opportunity has not been taken to build strong relationships with those few key decision makers. Wandering the halls of the executive suite and getting yourself known becomes particularly challenging when you consider that often the project leader must interact with executives who reside at different locations around the world. Even so, this important initiative is a high priority activity.

A successful project leader must consistently be actively involved in the process when key project presentations are being made to management or when key project decisions need to be taken. This is of fundamental importance because of the need to send an important message to the organization that the project leader is the key project spokesman and also one of the few individuals in the entire organization who can provide a balanced, informed, and impartial perspective on project issues.

Having the opportunity and responsibility to deal with senior management also means that a project leader must be sensitive to the needs of many individuals in positions of management responsibility and who need to be kept "in the loop" on key project activities. These individuals, particularly functional department heads, should be given the opportunity to support the team process as partners and should be encouraged by the project leader to provide assistance to the team when it is desired and necessary. The project leader must be careful not to build up walls between the project leader and these key individuals but instead must "reach out" and take the first step in developing appropriate relationships with these key decision makers. This is particularly appropriate when issues arise which directly affect a department's performance or the scope of a department head's authority and responsibility (see Fig. 1).

A project leader will often appear in front of management groups at critical times during the development of a drug. The project leader must confidently and convincingly present the project's progress, issues, problems, and recommended solutions and on occasion must be prepared to stand up to some intense grilling. Those who might be intimidated by others in positions of power are not successful in this role. Senior management's tolerance for getting to the bottom line can often be short. A successful leader must see through the maze of complex issues and problems and articulate the "big picture" quickly and coherently to very busy senior executives. Often the team's proposals may not at first be in line with the stated or perceived position of management. Here again the project leader must have the fortitude and confidence to participate in constructive debate with senior management to convince them of the merits of the team's position. It would be unacceptable if the project leader just accepted management's

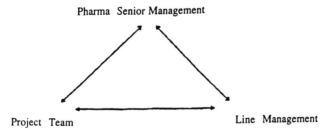

FIG. 1 Managing communication strategy to ensure timely, focused, and relevant exchange of information to the right customer groups is one of the most critical responsibilities of the project leader.

decision because "that is what management wanted" without first attempting to involve them in dialogue regarding the team's recommendations and rationale; this is one of the key responsibilities of the job.

B. Selecting the Right Team Leaders and the Right Team Members

Managing an international project team successfully starts with the organization of that team and with the characteristics and behavior expected of all team members, including the team leader. Setting expectations "up front" in terms of how team members are chosen and how the team is organized, the team members' individual roles and responsibilities, the team operating procedures, and the degree of decision making, authority, and autonomy expected of everyone are key elements for success.

1. Team Leaders

When evaluating candidates for the position of international project leader, there are a number of personal dimensions and prior job experiences which should be considered. With the cost of developing a new chemical entity exceeding $300 million and with mounting external and internal pressures on organizations to develop these compounds as rapidly and as cost effectively as possible, companies turn first to individuals with a great deal of drug development experience who know how to navigate their way through the myriad activities required to develop a new drug. Although drug development experience is clearly an important asset, organizations value more highly those individuals with the intellectual and intuitive capacities to understand complex issues, and those who can direct activities falling within and between the many disciplines represented on the project team, particularly those disciplines where the project leader is expert.

A project leader must manage a team where team members come from diverse cultural and educational backgrounds, with varying degrees of expertise, experience, and competence, and are located at different sites around the world. Given the complexity of drug development and the logistical and management challenges presented, one individual cannot know all the details of every aspect of a project. Even so, a project leader must still find the time and a way to control the project, know or have a sense of what is going on, and ensure that progress is being made and that project goals and time lines are achieved as scheduled. Although it is difficult to step back from project details, particularly when problems develop which require immediate resolution and which could benefit from management intervention, a project leader must resist the temptation to jump into every fray. Getting involved too often and too deeply in the internal workings of any one specific department, especially in a department where the project leader already has a great deal of experience, means that the leader will almost definitely not have sufficient time to manage the entire project effectively. A successful project leader must learn through experience when it is appropriate to become personally involved in a particular issue and what issues are worth becoming involved in to ensure prompt resolution of the more important issues and problems.

The discipline of project management in many companies has evolved over the years from one primarily of project coordination to one of project leadership. With this change has also come a change in the educational background and experience required in the job. More than ever, organizations are looking for individuals who have advanced scientific degrees and who have spent considerable time in senior research positions. Provided with a strong scientific underpinning, a project leader is now expected to be able to dialogue intelligently with scientists peer to peer and to understand a broad range of scientific findings and issues. A cautionary warning, however, must be raised. Although proficiency in a scientific discipline is clearly an important asset, accepting the position of project leadership means that an individual must have the discipline to focus on running the project and managing the scientists on the project, not doing the science. A project leader must maintain a broad and impartial perspective on issues, regardless of whether they emanate from scientific, technical, or commercial disciplines, and must allow and, more importantly, encourage the team members to solve their own problems and take responsibility for their own tasks. It is more important for the leader to ask the "right question" at the "right time" than trying to come up with the "right answer" personally. Being proficient as a generalist will serve the project leader well and will certainly provide more benefit to the team process than focusing effort on being the resident expert.

The successful project leader imparts vision to the team and instills enthusiasm and commitment in all team members to achieve a common goal. Providing vision in an effective manner certainly consists of clearly enumerating the direction, goals, and values the project leader expects all team members to embrace. To obtain commitment, however, each team member must be appropriately supported in successfully carrying out his agreed upon responsibilities.

A project leader's performance is constantly being judged by others within the organization and the ability to "walk the talk" is a critical component of daily life. Team members must feel comfortable working in a multidisciplinary team environment and to a great extent the leader is responsible for doing everything possible to create a positive atmosphere of teamwork and trust within the team to facilitate project ownership by all team members. On occasion, the position of project leadership is a lightning rod for senior management as they look for an outlet to vent their frustrations when things go astray during the long drug development process. Under these circumstances, it might be fairly easy for a project leader to pass the buck to someone else, particularly if the reason for management's frustration can be traced to a miscalculation or oversight by one of the team members. It is important, however, that the leader avoid the temptation to "point fingers" and instead share responsibility collectively with the team.

This does not mean that a project leader covers up improper or inexcusable actions or decision making; it does mean, however, striving to create an enthusiastic and productive team environment where team members experience the support provided by the project leader and are encouraged to support one another, even under adverse or uncomfortable circumstances.

The successful leader is the individual who basks in the accomplishments of others and in fact goes out of the way to ensure proper recognition of all team members, particularly when significant project accomplishments or milestones are achieved. A key working tenet should be that if any one team member is successful, then as a consequence the whole team including the project leader is also successful; it is inappropriate that all positive attention is directed to the project leader.

Another important characteristic of a successful project leader is the ability to accept criticism constructively and to maturely use feedback from others as input to improve personal performance. This is not always easy to do. It is understandable to rationalize away personal criticism as not being justified or feeling that this kind of input is misdirected and should more appropriately be focused on someone else. This, however, is not productive and the leader must possess the courage and maturity to honestly evaluate the source and basis of the personal criticism and decide whether or not to implement any changes in behavior as a result of the comments.

There are times during the development process when a project leader must dissociate from the project and objectively assess whether or not the project's value still justifies being kept in the portfolio. Being an advocate for a project is certainly admirable. However, this must be done responsibly. When it is time to assess a project's worth, the project leader must ensure that the team is as prepared as possible with all the relevant facts and data.

There may be team members and others within the organization who want to perform "that additional experiment" or request that more analyses be generated before critical project decisions are taken. Sometimes these requests are generated because of an honest feeling that insufficient data are available to make an appropriate decision, but sometimes these requests are motivated by a desire just to keep a project alive. The project leader must balance the need for more data which could result in better decision making with the need to make project decisions more rapidly. If a project no longer has what it takes to stay in the portfolio, then the project leader has a responsibility to the organization to make this recommendation and not let that judgment be colored by anyone's years of involvement with the project.

A project leader often takes on the role of the responsible cheerleader on the team, on one hand, to motivate team members when things do not go as planned, and on the other hand, to ensure that the team does not become too euphoric when things go better than anticipated. Teams go through significant emotional highs and lows throughout the development process. It is important for the leader to realize that things are never as good as they seem nor as bad as they are and that everyone's emotions are kept within a reasonable balance. The project leader must ensure that the team's enthusiasm does not influence their project objectivity, either positively or negatively. The successful leader should honestly utilize different leadership styles, depending on the situation presented, to influence other people's behavior throughout the development process. "Different strokes for different folks" works. With this in mind, the project leader must be particularly sensitive to individual circumstances, personalities, and needs.

The position of project leadership is an extremely taxing one and becomes even more stressful when facing the challenge of managing an international team. The project leader must be flexible and adaptable in a constantly changing and challenging environment, must provide leadership to others, and display significant personal and professional initiative. There are times when this individual must be aggressive and confidently challenge the status quo without being negatively confrontational, and there are other times when a more passive role is required to achieve objectives.

2. Team Members

Although team members have certain expectations of the project leader, the leader also has certain expectations of team members. A project leader expects that each team member is prepared with sufficient functional expertise and experience to provide an appropriate assessment and interpretation of data which the member or member's department has generated and to actively participate in the team's discussion and decision making process. In addition, the leader must assume and should expect that each team member will be empowered by the member's department to commit sufficient resources required to conduct and complete any planned studies in the time frames which have been agreed to. Team members are responsible for interacting with their functional manager to ensure departmental support and the prior commitment and availability of any requested and agreed upon financial and human resources.

It would be ideal if every member of every project team had prior project-related experience and was quite senior within the member's department. The problem often faced, however, is that there are not enough experienced people to cover all projects and, as a result, some project leaders find that they must deal with relatively inexperienced and junior team members. Under these circumstances, the leader must insist that the individual department functions take on the added responsibility to provide training and coaching for their own team representatives to get them up to speed as rapidly as possible and that senior members within these departments are active in mentoring younger colleagues. Unfortunately, this is not always done within the function and it is often expected that somehow the project leader addresses these deficiencies. Until such time that team members represent their departments appropriately and establish a level of credibility within their own organization, the project leader faces the problem of a somewhat dysfunctional team where some team members disregard or dismiss what others have to say primarily because of a lack of confidence in these "junior members." This situation must be addressed as rapidly as possible by the project leader and the functional manager working in concert.

A project leader who has been around for some time in an organization usually knows who in the various departments are the good performers and who are the ones to avoid. Of course, from a selfish perspective, leaders feel that their project is the most important in the entire portfolio and want only the best performers or those the leaders are most comfortable with on the project team. Unfortunately, every project leader usually winds up wanting the same individuals, so internal competition develops as individuals attempt to stack the deck or "cherry pick" the organization with these "winners." The functional manager then has the difficult task of deciding who from his department goes on which project team. This usually winds up as a "win-lose" situation and certainly is a negative experience. This competitive process must be carefully managed by all participants. Ground rules must be agreed upon beforehand so that there are no surprises or misunderstandings.

Because of the small size of some departments and the lack of sufficient numbers of qualified individuals within departments, many managers wind up assigning one person to more than one project team. This is certainly expedient from the perspective of the department head, in fact, there may be no other option. However, this could be quite problematic from the perspective of the project leader and makes it difficult to build a well-functioning and aligned project team. It is unfair to expect that individuals feels completely part of any one team if there are conflicting demands on their time and energy from two or more teams and project leaders. While there may be little that an individual project leader can do to resolve this situation, the leader must ensure that, at least in those few key departments critical to the project's success, appropriate team representation and sufficient resources and attention are provided. Depending upon the tasks which need to be completed, this may or may not require the full-time commitment of some individuals within the organization.

There is significant partnering required between the project leader and the functional manager on many issues, including the fact that both must work together to ensure that the performance of individual team members consistently meet high standards. This means that communications between these two individuals must be frequent, and often times brutally honest. Of course there are organizational barriers which must be overcome and prior relationships which may make this difficult to achieve. It may not be easy for the functional manager to completely understand or accept the role and position of the project leader. This is particularly difficult when the scope and extent of the functional manager's work experience has been within a traditional line organization with defined reporting relationships and responsibilities, whereas the project leader's role is substantially focused on the interaction and interrelationships within a matrix environment (see Fig. 2).

Besides expecting individual functional expertise and project experience, it is also absolutely critical for the project leader to expect and demand that every team member perform appropriately as a team player. This is no small task given the fact that often times individuals are hired into organizations primarily for their expertise and not for their ability to work well on a team. Prima donnas, even with strong scientific expertise and considered critical to a project, are quite destructive to the team process and certainly make it difficult for the leader to successfully manage the team. This issue must be addressed quickly and firmly and should be accepted as a shared responsibility between the project leader and the functional manager who need to work in concert to address issues of individual behavior and attitude.

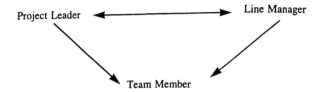

FIG. 2 The project leader and functional manager share responsibility in managing the performance of a team member. These two executives must align themselves and ensure that their individual efforts support one another.

Choosing who in the function deserves and merits being on a project team becomes a very important decision for the organization. Although the ultimate responsibility for appointing team members resides primarily within the function and must be the primary responsibility of the functional manager, it is critical that the project leader also play a role in this process and provide input before final decisions are made. If concerns need to be raised about the appointment of a team member because of past performance or personal reasons, it is better that these concerns are raised before the individual is appointed to a project team. A responsible project leader must make performance expectations known and not compromise the high standards demanded from everyone, including the leader.

Although the size of a project team varies widely, it usually ranges between 10 to 20 team members. Despite its size, however, there are usually only a few individuals on the team who wind up as the key project "drivers." Most often these individuals come from the clinical, marketing, and regulatory departments. The leader must cultivate special relationships with these individuals because of the need to rely more on this small group than on others on the team. Particular attention must be paid so that this core group is aligned and agrees on key strategic initiatives and on those critical project decisions which significantly affect the project's future success. Although the project leader should pay particular attention to these team members, other members of the team must not be alienated and wind up creating a two-tier system of "haves" and "have nots." All members of the project team are and must feel that they are contributors to the team process, that their opinions are valued, and that they can and are in fact encouraged to participate actively during team discussion and decision making.

Decisions regarding the most appropriate site locations for key project team members are also critical in setting up an international project team and are fundamental to its operation. These decisions are most appropriately made after the roles, responsibilities, and expectations of the team and team members have been agreed to by management and ideally should involve the project leader along with key functional managers and representatives from senior management. Although these decisions are influenced by where the functional therapeutic expertise may reside, having at least the core team members at one location is the preferred alternative.

There is no one way to effectively configure a team. One approach would be for all team members to reside in one location. Although this minimizes many of the communication issues which often arise in managing an international project team, the team must be aware that it lacks the full appreciation for and knowledge of regulatory and marketing issues at other sites. This deficiency must be appreciated and more importantly, must be addressed. A great deal of responsibility to ensure that the needs of worldwide markets are appropriately balanced and considered, before key project decisions are made, falls primarily on the shoulders of the project leader who is expected to have the broadest impartial project perspective. Conversely, if team members reside at various locations around the world, information about local or regional requirements must become more accessible and transparent to all team members. However, communication issues now become more problematic. Here again the leader must take on the added responsibility to establish appropriate mechanisms and procedures for minimizing communication roadblocks which arise.

C. Team Goals and Team Commitment

Besides monitoring an individual team member's performance to maximize the team process, team goals and objectives must be carefully negotiated and agreed to and performance metrics must be tied to appropriate and acceptable reward systems. In managing an international project team, personal involvement in setting objectives is one of the more important duties of the project leader. The fact that team members often reside in different locations and are subject to different compensation systems certainly makes this a difficult task; even so, within the constraints of local customs and regulations, the project leader needs to ensure an equitable reward system for project performance.

As a project moves through development, the project leader must ensure that the individual and collective plans and contributions of all team members are aligned and support the project's key strategies and tactics which have been agreed to. To accomplish this effectively, it is paramount that, every year, individual and team performance goals which are SMART (specific, measurable, attainable, results oriented, and time bound) be negotiated and agreed to within the team and ultimately with management. Project goal setting should be a formalized process encouraged and embraced by the organization. The first step is taken by the team and results in setting those few critical team goals (usually 4 to 6) which, if appropriately and successfully addressed, have a major impact on the project's progress during the year or significantly affect prospects for approvability and/or marketability. Every member of the team should have the opportunity to participate in this process, and, within the team setting, debate and negotiate those goals felt most important.

Each team member must also share collective responsibility for the team's commitments to the organization. This is a key issue, for at the end of the year, an individual's performance assessment also reflects whether or not the team's goals have been met. Often times this is quite a problematic issue, particularly if a team member feels able to contribute only minimally, if at all, to the achievement of a particular goal and that the member's own performance is measured by the line function on the achievement of the departmental objectives for which the individual is responsible. If, for example, a team decides that one of its key goals is developing a publication plan, a quality control chemist might feel somewhat uncomfortable having his overall performance judged by whether or not this "marketing activity" is completed on time. If, however, the team is to "own its own project," then all team members must share responsibility in owning these goals which are felt by the team to be most important to the project's success. The project leader must ensure that every team member understands this important principle.

Team goals often are activity-based initiatives or outcomes which are fairly easy to articulate and measure, i.e., reaching a specific milestone by a certain date, publishing results in a particular journal, or developing a specific plan of action within a projected time frame. However, team goals also reflect how well the team is working together. For example, are team problems being resolved effectively in "win-win" situations? How is information being shared within a project? Are team members supportive of one another? These "softer" goals tend to be overlooked, but they are extremely important and reflect attitudes and behavior which, if not properly managed by the project leader, influence whether the team meets its more activity-based goals.

Once team goals have been agreed to, the team has a framework within which it can operate and a reference point against which its performance (as a team) can be measured. In addition, team members also have the opportunity to develop their own individual goals within this framework in which they can tie their individual goals to the team goals and ensure that their own goals do not conflict with those proposed by other team members. Sharing of individual goals within the team is a critical activity enabling each team member to know what others are planning and helping avoid situations where conflicting expectations arise over the projected availability of key project "deliverables" throughout the year. This is an important part of the overall process and as such needs the active involvement of the project leader to ensure optimal collaboration and coordination among all team members.

It would be extremely productive if the project leader took the time to meet with each team member to review individual project goals and objectives and to ensure agreement with what is being proposed. The project leader must be confident that these goals also have the support of management and that the requisite resources are committed so that each team member successfully completes the agreed upon tasks as scheduled. If required, discussion about individual goals and target dates can certainly involve the team member, project leader, and functional manager. However, it is usually preferable that the team member first reach agreement with his own management so that particularly sensitive department-related issues and problems are discussed and resolved within the function (see Fig. 3).

1. Meeting Aggressive Time Lines

A key challenge which the project leader must address is the often expressed concern that target dates once committed become "etched in stone." During the normal course of drug development, new scientific findings often arise which require initiating additional unplanned studies or spending additional time understanding study findings. Many believe that management is often reluctant to change dates once they are agreed to, despite apparent

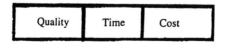

FIG. 3   The achievement of individual and team goals must result in tangible deliverables which move a project forward. All goals are built on basic project tenets of high quality output, rapid time to market development, and responsible cost management.

changes in the internal or external project environment. Based on these perceptions, team members are often reluctant to project aggressive target dates for completing their project goals and build slack into their time lines to plan for the unexpected and to successfully meet their commitments. To avoid creating or supporting an environment where team members consistently "pad their project," the project leader must be aware of potential project risks and individual team member's concerns. It is useful to ensure that interim target dates for key project goals are provided to allow the team to reevaluate its commitments to management on an ongoing basis. When and if significant findings occur which require program modification, then the project leader has information available early enough which he can present to management to negotiate agreement with any justifiable changes in time lines which are proposed.

Teams and individuals are continually being challenged and encouraged to stretch their goals to push their projects as aggressively as possible. Although realistic target goals are often utilized to evaluate team performance, teams are also asked to bracket their goals with sets of assumptions to project optimistic and pessimistic targets as well. The project leader must ensure that team members take on this challenge constructively and stretch themselves to think "out of the box" by providing responsible best and worst case scenarios. Of course, if the team achieves its optimistic targets, then their rewards should be commensurate with their achievements. The project leader must be able to negotiate reward systems ahead of time to provide appropriate recognition for optimal performance.

When setting multiple targets, i.e., optimistic, realistic, and pessimistic completion dates for key activities, the critical question that needs to be resolved is On what basis do you reward accomplishments? Clearly, if an optimistic target is achieved, teams should receive the maximum reward possible. However, should teams be rewarded to a greater extent when an optimistic target date is missed or when a realistic date is achieved? One could argue that the former is more important to the organization because it is likely to result in completing a particular goal at an earlier date. Whatever the approach, it is critical to create an environment where teams and team members do not feel that they have failed because they have missed a target date. Unless managed properly, however, an individual's fear of failure can cause padding in a target date to ensure that the date is met. The project leader must be a champion within his own organization to support a philosophy that goals need to be set aggressively and that, if dates are missed, individuals are not "punished." When target dates are missed, it is the responsibility of all members of the organization to collectively examine those systems and processes which prevented the team from meeting its goals. Organizations should learn from experience, and, if they embrace the philosophy that systems and processes constantly need improvement and are the likely reason why the team did not meet its goal, then the next team facing similar challenges might indeed be successful.

2. Budgetary Responsibility

The project leader must also create an environment where team members approach their everyday challenges as if they were working for themselves. Team members need to remain focused on doing a quality job in the shortest period of time, and they also must pay particular attention to completing their tasks within an agreed budget or allowed budget variance (i.e., ±5% or ±10%). If a team is to "own" its project, the team must feel that it has responsibility for and some control over the money that is committed and spent. The team has a fiduciary responsibility and as such also needs to set yearly budget targets against which their performance is measured. Although budget control normally is a responsibility of the line function, the team must play a role in setting budget targets based on planned project activities. The project leader must ensure that the team has the tools available within the organization to appropriately track budget performance and assure that expenditures are proper and that appropriate controlling action is taken when budget variances occur. The project leader should negotiate an allowance with senior management for a reasonable discretionary budget which can be managed and utilized by the team to support unanticipated activities which need to be initiated during the year. In addition, to further support team responsibility and ownership, if there are budget overruns on some project activities, it is appropriate to provide the team with the flexibility to "move money around the project" themselves without obtaining management approval; this builds project ownership.

Budgets are usually developed and managed locally with responsibility under the aegis of department heads who are accountable to their own line management for keeping expenses within an agreed upon target. These managers are often confronted with requests to support a multitude of project team initiatives, i.e., international travel for a team member to visit another site, travel for presentations at symposia, meetings with regulatory authorities at various locations throughout the world, etc., some of which may have been previously planned and some of which arise unexpectedly during the year. To control department expenses which may already be stretched to the limit, particularly toward the end of the budget year, a functional manager often takes the position that his budget cannot support the team's request and that funds must be provided by the project leader or by the project team. However, unless sufficient funds are previously allocated to the project leader for such contingencies, the team's request is not accommodated and intervention and resolution are needed from senior management. Although these situations cannot always be avoided, if the team's request is critical in supporting the achievement of already agreed to project goals, it is likely that management will support these budget overruns. The position often and appropriately taken by management is that "the project comes first, the budget second." Of course, this is relevant only as long as the project leader and project team first demonstrate a degree of fiduciary responsibility in running their project.

3. Reward and Recognition

Linking rewards to the achievement of key project goals also encourages team members to focus their efforts primarily on those activities which support the more important project strategies and tactics. This also instills a sense of urgency and appreciation that "time means money," especially to those individuals on the team who significantly affect the project's outcome. Assuming that the project leader has negotiated a reasonable and responsible reward and recognition system, now there is an additional tool available to help manage the team successfully. However, when considering rewards and recognition, the project leader must expand his focus beyond the project team and acknowledge that there are many other individuals within every function who are also critical in contributing to a project's success.

For example, the toxicologist on the project team cannot meet time commitments if the pathologist or lab technician or secretary within Toxicology do not complete their own tasks as scheduled; the clinical leader needs the statistician, the data manager, the Clinical Research Associate and others to help implement the clinical program effectively; etc. Every team member has a "shadow" team behind him which must perform well and is aligned with the overall goals and timetables of the project team. If this can be accomplished, the development process is usually a smooth one. However, if the team is successful in achieving its goals, how do you equitably reward all those critical people who are not part of the project team? This is not an easy issue to resolve and certainly points to one of the many difficulties inherent in any reward and recognition system, i.e., Who is eligible and what system fairly recognizes all those individuals without whom the project goals are not met? Although resolution of this issue does not fall under the direct purview of the project leader, this is a potential problem and the negative consequences of championing the rewarding of some individuals, results in disappointing others who could feel particularly slighted.

When evaluating individual performance, the project leader should request input from other core team members before reaching his final assessment and recommendation. By sharing this important responsibility, the project leader can more fairly provide balanced and objective input and minimize any personal bias which might influence the evaluation of team members. It is critical to the successful management of an international project team that the project leader's recommendations are considered seriously by the functional manager before the employee's overall yearly performance evaluation is finalized. This process must be encouraged and supported by senior management. While assessing individual performance and achievement at the end of every year is reasonably accomplished, it is much more difficult at key milestones or at the end of a project when you want to assign special bonuses to individuals. How, for example, do you evaluate and reward the performance and impact of someone who has been on a project for a number of years with a colleague who has only been on a project for less than one year? Assuming equal performance, it is fair to reward the former more than the latter. To equitably accomplish this, a performance grid is recommended as a tool for the project leader. See the example below of project performance/years on a project.

	Recommended Bonus		
Rating	<1 year	1–3 years	>3 years
Superior	6%	8%	10%
Excellent	4%	6%	8%
Very Good	2%	4%	6%

Of course, to send the right message to the organization, care must be taken to reward the better performers significantly more than the average performers. Consistent with setting aggressive team and individual goals, average performance does not deserve special recognition. In addition, the project leader needs to be aware that individuals, who at one time contributed significantly to the project and who are now reassigned to other responsibilities, should not be forgotten, for they too deserve reward and recognition.

D. Project Planning

The project leader needs to ensure that project plans are well thought out, transparent to the organization, aggressive in time-to-market projections, have the backing of the various functional departments, and, if successful, support the achievement of the desired target profile/package insert.

By utilizing appropriate planning and control systems in his project, the successful project leader demonstrates leadership capability and creates and manages a myriad of mechanisms critical to the project leader and team throughout the drug development process. It is critical that, whatever tools are agreed upon to accomplish this objective, they are user friendly, useful to the project leader and the project team, and accessible to and used by all members of the team and others in the organization. It is anticipated and expected that these tools enable the team to develop integrated and aggressive project development plans with appropriate intermediate milestones and also ensure that the planning process is thorough enough to avoid downtime between critical path activities.

Project plans and schedules, which can be agreed upon, are critical prerequisites for obtaining individual commitments on projects. The project leader, team member, and functional manager must collectively know what tasks are committed to and when functional resources are required to perform and complete tasks as scheduled. For those individuals involved, progress on project plans must be appropriately monitored so that individual team members do not feel that their every working moment is being scrutinized by their organization. In addition, plans and schedule changes must be communicated to the organization periodically to ensure that all contributors stay aligned with project goals and performance expectations. Changes do indeed occur throughout development; it is imperative therefore that the project leader quickly communicate program modifications so that there are no unexpected surprises or misunderstandings with those whose commitments are affected by these changes.

To effectively lead a team, the team leader should be comfortable with and proficient in various planning, scheduling, and monitoring procedures and with mechanisms for developing budget estimates and control procedures. Project control is achieved in various ways, i.e., by setting mutually agreed objectives and goals, defining the various tasks which need to be performed, scheduling the tasks in concert with the functional departments in terms of resource requirements and availability, measuring project progress and performance in a clear, unbiased, and transparent manner, taking corrective action when progress is not made or when things do not go as planned, resolving conflicts as appropriate or raising them in a professional manner to higher management levels for appropriate resolution, etc.

A sound, responsible, and agreed upon project plan, developed early in the development process, which supports the agreed target profile and is "revisited" periodically throughout the development process to ensure that it reflects the latest project status and best thinking of the team, is extremely important to a project's ultimate success and is a critical tool for the successful project leader and the international project team. This plan must reflect the most appropriate road map so that the corporation can maximize its return on investment. An integral part of this planning process, therefore, must be the early development of an agreed upon package insert, highlighting particularly those claims and attributes which are key for successful marketing. Based on these claims, the design of critical clinical studies can be focused to generate the relevant data.

Every team member must be involved in building the project plan. Measurable milestones must be defined against which team performance is assessed. In addition, mechanisms must be agreed to which allow detecting problems early enough, so that solutions are found to keep the project on track.

Project management techniques, such as PERT planning and critical path analysis, provide the project leader with the information required to stay on top of his project. For these tools to be most useful, however, all team members should have access to the same information as the project leader so that they understand where their "piece of the puzzle" fits and, more importantly, how well they and their team members are doing compared to the commitments that have been made. These planning techniques allow all project tasks to be optimally integrated and reduce project task duration through reduced overlapping of key activities, simulation modeling, and evaluation of contingency alternatives.

1. Project Team Meetings

Meetings that are not well planned and well run are significant time wasters, serve little useful purpose, are a financial burden to the organization, and pose problems for the project leader in effectively synergizing interactions between team members and motivating them to meet high performance standards.

Often most people in an organization feel that there is insufficient quality time during the day to accomplish their daily objectives. Acknowledging and respecting this frustrating problem, the project leader's time must be managed as productively as possible, and as the leader of a team, an environment must be created where others have the opportunity to manage and use their own time effectively as well. Because of the problem of long distances between the sites of team members who are on international project teams and need to come together and communicate frequently, significant time usually must be committed to attending team meetings. For these meetings to be worthwhile, the meeting outcomes must result in tangible "deliverables" and the team must feel that the time spent together has been productive and has helped move their project forward. As examples of expected outcomes, it must be obvious that decisions have been taken, that issues have been resolved, that data have been shared, and that "added value" has been achieved.

Developing a detailed agenda sent to team members sufficiently in advance of each meeting to provide time to adequately prepare for the team's discussion, is one of the prerequisites for ensuring a focused and successful meeting. Every agenda item must identify the key individual or individuals who are the primary stakeholders and who are most responsible to lead the particular discussion, must clearly spell out the reasons why the item is even on the agenda (i.e., a problem statement), and must enumerate the outcome expected from the team's discussion. Given sufficient notice, team members have no excuse for coming poorly prepared to team meetings. If this occurs, it signals a problematic issue for the project leader because a lack of preparedness means a lack of commitment to the team process and team working agreements and, as such, must be addressed and resolved quickly and firmly.

2. Team Dynamics

Although open and constructive debate, which seeks and encourages input from all team members, is important to consensus building, the project leader, more often than not, should first identify and then resolve extremely contentious and/or personnel issues apart from and prior to the team meeting. If this is not done, and particularly if it is apparent that the issue under debate is important to only a few individuals, the whole team becomes captive to an uncomfortable discussion that usually drags on as the "combatants" battle out their differences, usually without resolution and with an expected "lose-lose" outcome. If the project leader feels that a particular issue is likely to evoke a great deal of emotion, it is prudent to consider a pre-meeting meeting where those few team members, who are primarily involved, can come together to cool things down and sort out their differences in a nonthreatening, private, and hopefully productive environment. Sufficient agreement on at least a portion of the issue must be reached and the issue already defused before a "core agreed position" is brought forward to the whole team.

During the conduct of team meetings, it is sometimes observed that a few individuals, either because of their personalities or their positions or both, dominate the discussion, usually to the detriment of other, more reticent team members. Although the project leader is responsible for allowing all individuals sufficient "air time" to fairly present their cases and provide their perspective, the project leader is the gate keeper of available time and must gently but firmly redirect the discussion to provide an opportunity for other team members to contribute their opinions as well. Handling this situation must be done somewhat delicately, particularly since some individuals find it difficult to cogently articulate their feelings in a team setting. Often, their reasons appear quite valid, at least to the team members, i.e., they might be shy, they might be junior members of the team, they might not want to go up against what appears to be the growing team consensus, or even worse, they might feel that the project leader has abrogated responsibility and given up control of the discussion allowing a free-for-all with clear winners and losers. It is critical to ensure that, during the team meeting, the discussion is open and factual and is not allowed to drift too far from the agenda item, that a good exchange of opinion is allowed and even encouraged, particularly if there are dissenting views, and that the project leader not permit the discussion to degrade to a level of personal attack between team members.

To accomplish this, the project leader must concentrate efforts to ensure that the dynamics of the meeting run smoothly and be aware of the verbal and nonverbal signals that are sent. Of course, while concentrating efforts on running the meeting and keeping a pulse on the meeting dynamics, the project leader must also accurately capture the myriad of key meeting outcomes which need to be shared with the organization, i.e., problems which have been identified, solutions which have been recommended, decisions which have been taken, dissenting opinions, agreed to next steps and milestones, individual responsibilities, timetables, etc. Quite a monumental task. Either the project leader takes minutes of the meeting or preferably requests that a team member serve as the meeting secretary. If the latter approach is agreed to by the team, the project leader should insist that this task is shared on a rotating basis by all team members.

It is absolutely critical that team meetings begin and finish on time so that team members can get on with their other tasks and duties. The project leader must be alert to and avoid situations where individuals stroll into a scheduled meeting five or ten minutes after it has started; this is certainly disruptive to the meeting process. These same individuals would never think twice about arriving ten minutes late for an appointment with the president of the company. Then why should their tardiness to a team meeting be expected or, even worse, tolerated? If the project leader delays the scheduled start of a meeting until all team members have arrived, the wrong signal is sent to the whole team and particularly to those members of the team who are sitting at the table waiting for the meeting to start. If this occurs, then the next time the project leader calls a meeting, even more team members will stroll in late. It is of utmost importance therefore to set critical meeting expectations and agree ahead of time on "team standard operating procedures" regarding meeting conduct and participation. If some members habitually come late to meetings, the project manager must resolve this issue immediately and not let it linger. If resolution cannot be achieved, then this issue must be escalated up the chain of command.

3. Meeting Documentation

To avoid any misunderstandings, at the conclusion of the meeting, the project leader takes a few minutes to summarize the key agreements and action steps and to reiterate those issues which still need to be resolved. Every team member should walk away from the meeting with the same understanding of what occurred. Therefore, by briefly reviewing the meeting highlights, the project leader drives home the key meeting messages to everyone. All critical project information must be communicated to the organization in a timely manner. It should be a clear team expectation that minutes are distributed no later than one week after the meeting. These minutes must be accurate, and they must highlight the critical issues and decisions that were made. To ensure accuracy, minutes are first sent to the meeting attendees for their review and comment. Sending out minutes for review does not mean that team members have the liberty to change what was agreed to at the meeting. This sometimes becomes an issue, particularly when team members are concerned with the way their functions might view the statements made during the meeting or are concerned that functional managers might not agree with the decisions made. The project leader is responsible to the entire team to ensure that, when minutes are finalized and distributed, they truly represent what actually happened at the meeting.

Besides ensuring accuracy, the project leader must also ensure readability, particularly when a great deal of information is being communicated. A one page summary should be attached to the minutes to succinctly highlight milestones achieved, critical issues, decisions made, follow-up actions, and time lines and individuals responsible for these actions. This short summary means that anyone receiving the minutes at least reads the highlights. For those interested in the details, they can and certainly will read the entire document.

6

Managing Joint Ventures

Building on Positives and the Effective Use of Project Management Techniques

David A. Dworaczyk

Solvay Pharmaceuticals, Inc.
Marietta, Georgia

I. CHAPTER SYNOPSIS AND INTRODUCTION

In our current world of industrial competitiveness, health care reform, government intervention, price controls, cost containment, company downsizing, budget restrictions, and the need to discover, develop, and market new and innovative products, the pressures facing many health care/pharmaceutical companies today are considerably different than they were even five years ago. Based on the fact that we cannot do business as we did in the past, many companies have explored new ways to find new products and generate income.

Historically, our industry has benefited from unusually high profitability and little intervention from outside sources. Based on this favorable environment, we were free to set and raise prices without much outside interference and to invest heavily in internal R&D efforts. Now, more than ever, there is increasing internal pressure to increase R&D productivity. This can be done in many ways, such as enhancing or increasing the level of internal effort. Or one can look outside the organization via licensing, acquisition, or partnering via formation of joint ventures or strategic alliances.

This particular chapter focuses on managing outside R&D alliances, partnerships, and joint ventures. There are numerous aspects of any outside venture that need to be considered from a business perspective, and these will only be touched upon here. The emphasis will be focused on R&D alliances/joint ventures, what to look for in establishing those relationships, and how to manage them once they are established. In this chapter, I will be using the analogy to marriage. Hopefully, many of you will understand the nuances of the analogy.

II. A GENERAL OVERVIEW OF ALLIANCES/JOINT VENTURES

Before we start, one point needs to be clear from the beginning, and that is that all alliance deals are unique. No two deals are exactly alike, nor should they be. There are commonalities, but each one is specific to the companies and/or product(s) in question. However, regardless of the deal pursued, there are several common activities/steps that should be taken when moving toward an alliance or joint venture (see Table 1).

Overall, each alliance or joint venture is a unique entity with its own approach toward fulfilling both partners' specific needs. However, R&D alliances/joint ventures can be generally classified into several categories, such as

A. Enabling Technologies: In these alliances, one partner is looking for a technology or expertise to complement its own internal efforts. The other partner supplies that tool. Examples of enabling technologies sought are

- combinatorial chemistry
- high-throughput pharmacological screening
- genetic positional cloning
- genetic mapping
- functional genomics
- gene biochemical pathway elucidation/expression.

B. Codevelopment: In these situations, one partner brings a new potential product into the alliance/joint venture and both partners provide the development resources (money, expertise, people, operational resources, etc.) to bring the product to the market.

C. Opportunistic Synergies: Unlike the examples noted above, in these cases, there is a concerted effort on the part of a single company to surround itself with numerous companies with varying and potentially complementary

TABLE 1

Steps to Building and Making an Alliance Work

1. Define your own internal development and/or growth strategy	• Know what you are • Know where you are now • Define where you want to be • Define what your organization can reasonably achieve and/or do • Define the time frame to achieve your goals
2. Identify your alternatives	• Identify all of the potential alternatives that you could pursue to achieve your goal • Evaluate those alternatives, and choose the one that has the greatest probability of success within your organization
3. If an alliance is the approach you are going to take, identify as many possible partners as possible	• Look for opportunities • Look for company, product, project and/or technology synergies or enhancements
4. Identify the best candidates, and then do the appropriate due diligence	• Find out as much as you can • Know your potential partners • Look for compatibility
5. Define alliance terms	• Operational • Commercial • Economic • Communication
6. Clearly define the project	• Who will do what when, where, and how • Define the milestones to monitor progress • Define decision criteria • Define how the project will be managed
7. Provide avenues for closure, escape, and/or continuance	• Define when the project is complete and how that will be determined • Provide an avenue for divergence and/or separation of the parties, if necessary • Insure that there is an opportunity to continue if it makes sense
8. Insure commitment and be ready to work	• Both parties must commit • Both parties must invest time, resources, and a desire to make the alliance work

technologies in the hope that, through effective integration and management of these different technologies, potential products are identified that are greater than the sum of their parts. In other words, through integrating multiple technologies from numerous alliances or ventures, new products can be identified that would not have been found without such an effort.

III. PERSONAL INTRODUCTIONS: INTERNAL AND EXTERNAL ASSESSMENTS OF BOTH YOURSELF AND YOUR POTENTIAL PARTNER

As in any personal relationships, which alliances and joint ventures are, it is important to know whom you are going to meet and also to know who you are. In most cases, there is often very little time spent in understanding who we are as companies and as individuals before we get into a "steamy affair." Let us not forget, we are after long-term relationships, not one-night stands. For long-term relationships to develop, there needs to be an aura of respect, openness, understanding, and trust. "One-night stands" are built mostly on blind passion and lust, which are hardly the qualities or emotions needed to sustain long-term relationships.

In many instances, companies follow a trend, rather than try to fully understand and visualize their goals, needs, expectations, capabilities, and capacities. This approach has led many organizations down a garden path that ends up in an unsightly divorce. These painful and/or costly experiences often lead to an aversion to try a new relationship, where in fact, mutual benefit could be realized.

Before any type of alliance or joint venture is pursued, it is important to address two basic questions: 1) What kind of a company are we?, and 2) What is our long-term vision and strategy?

To address the first question, it is helpful to take some time with the right people within your organization and address the following questions:

A. Do you have a clear vision of what the company will be? If so, does everyone understand it, buy into it and actively pursue it? Does everyone interpret the words to mean the same thing? Do your budgeting and planning activities move the company toward satisfying that vision, or are they short-term focused?

B. Is your company competing in a broad-based industry (e.g., health care), or is it focused (e.g., pharmaceuticals)?

C. Within that industry or industry segment, is it participating in the broadest markets or is it a niche player?

D. Where do you stand against your competitors in size (i.e., sales, budgets, R&D expenditure, people, number of products, customer base, etc.)?

E. What is the internal and external image/perception of your company held by your employees, customers, and competitors?

Answering these questions will provide you with a basis to begin looking at the next step in the internal assessment process, which is focusing on the second question mentioned above, What is your long-term strategy? A strategy can only follow from a clear vision and mission. Defining a strategy to fulfill a poorly thought through or too broad a vision will lead to disenchantment and demotivation of even your most dedicated employees and will, eventually, lead to failure. Unfortunately, rather than admit failure, many organizations abandon their strategy only to define another that is just as ambiguous and/or unobtainable rather than addressing the more fundamental issue of developing a clear and realistic mission and vision and, then, generating a realistic strategy from there.

Overall, there are five basic steps to developing a realistic strategy, assuming that the starting point is sound.

A. Assess where and what you are now.

B. Diagnose the reasons why you are what you are and where you are now. What are the factors, issues, restraints, capabilities, strengths, weaknesses, and actions that have created your organization of today?

Then, identify/develop

- what can reasonably be expected from your organization over the time frame of your strategy (i.e., current product sales, new product launches/sales, R&D output, etc.)
- the gap between where you want to be and what your organization can deliver
- realistic possible alternatives that can be put in place to fill the gap, and then, evaluate each of them, thoroughly, listing the risks and benefits of each, the probability of success of each, and the impact of closing the gap. In many cases, a multifaceted strategy will be developed because any one approach may not completely fill the gap between what you can reasonably achieve yourself and your goal.

C. Develop an action plan to implement the strategy.

D. Actually implement the strategy.

E. Reassess the outcomes/progress periodically to see if the strategy you have chosen is still the right one to pursue, if modifications are necessary, or if things are moving better than expected.

If one of the realistic alternatives identified is to pursue an alliance or joint venture, however, another party becomes part of and critical in your overall success, or failure. It will also have its own identity, vision, mission and strategy, which should be compatible and synergistic with yours, or at least can be adapted to help both parties achieve their long-term visions.

In all joint ventures and alliances, there is an implicit rule that is often forgotten or ignored and that is that both parties should feel that they are wanted, needed, trusted, respected, and will benefit from the joint venture/alliance. If either partner feels used, abused, or taken for granted, the partnership will fail. This effect can be minimized through an intense internal and an external assessment of your own organization and your potential partner's. There needs to be a clear understanding of who and what a company is, what it wants (i.e., goals and expectations), where it plans to go, along with when and how it plans to get there, before any external arrangement can be struck.

After there is a clear understanding of your own organization's goals, needs, and expectations, an active effort can be initiated to seek a partner which appears to be a good match. As in many personal relationships, a potential partner is often identified by visual cues, i.e., does the potential partner "look" attractive. However, if a short list of potential partners is developed based only on superficial characteristics, the chances of developing long-term relationships are significantly diminished. The potential for surprises, unknown habits, and/or the realization of cultural differences can and have destroyed more than one alliance.

The key to any long-term relationship is to really get to know your potential partner, know their parents, if there are any, as well as their brothers and sisters, i.e., know of other partners and their other relationships to determine if the partnership you are trying to strike would create a conflict at any level. Therefore, an in-depth review and assessment of all potential partners is essential. Hopefully, the following steps will help guide you through this process.

IV. DANCING: CORPORATE CHEMISTRY, THE SCIENCE OF COMPATIBILITY

The following are key factors, issues, and concerns that should be addressed early.

A. Know Yourself

Understand who and what your company is, what it wants, what its goals and expectations are, where it wants to go, and how long is it willing to wait to get there. It is absolutely essential to understand clearly what you see as the goals or objectives for proposing the option of forming an alliance. There may be commercial expectations, such as expanding an existing franchise, building one, or opening up a new geographic market (i.e., market expansion), or your corporate goals may be R&D focused, such as gaining new technology, expanding your R&D pipeline, entering a new therapeutic area, sharing development risk and cost, expanding expertise/know-how, or gaining more capacity to expedite development schedules.

In some cases, there may be senior managers who have their perception of "reality" based on their own individual assessment of the internal and external environments, regardless of accuracy or validity. If these individuals are open to discussion and input and are willing to perhaps change their positions through presentation of other views and/or information, then, there is a greater chance that a realistic view of the situation can be accepted. However, there is also a chance that their views may be confirmed, and this should also be readily accepted by all parties. In either case, it must be understood that a senior manager's or key stakeholder's perception of the situation may become reality.

Corporate goals or objectives must be clearly described and understood. Once the internal corporate goal(s) are clearly defined, then, various strategic options can be identified and evaluated in an attempt to select the one that will provide you with the greatest probability of achieving your goal.

It is important to define your options because there are many possible strategies that could be followed to achieve the defined corporate goal. An alliance or partnership, at any level, is only one approach. Although there may be some overlap in the reasons why a company chooses to pursue a merger or acquisition over building an alliance or partnership, strategic alliances, ventures, or partnerships are generally formed for long-term strategic reasons. It is fairly unlikely that an alliance or partnership will be a viable approach for a "quick fix" to any short-term problem. An alliance is a long-term affair. The organizational impact and financial gains, if any, will not be seen in the next quarterly financial report, but rather they will only be realized, in most cases, over a 5–15 year horizon, depending on the project involved.

Another issue to consider is an alliance may not decrease costs or reduce time. It is, generally, accepted that partnerships can provide advantages, such as reduced financial commitment, shared risk, and potentially greater flexibility (i.e., your own internal resources can be deployed to other projects). However, unless the alliance or partnership is created so that it provides a mechanism to develop, monitor, and work at and through these issues, prospectively, there is a good chance that an alliance or partnership will not provide you with the advantages sought.

An alliance also creates burdens that should not be overlooked. Successful alliances are true working partnerships. They involve strategic, operational, tactical, personal, personnel, and financial commitments. Your organization must understand the scope of the internal investment necessary to make partnerships work and be willing to providing these elements to the alliance for the long-term to realize the defined goals.

Another factor, often overlooked, is that there is no guarantee of success with an alliance. The probability of success can be increased substantially by addressing the points and issues described in this chapter, but nothing has a 100 percent guarantee. Therefore, even if an alliance is chosen as the path to take, it is prudent to develop a contingency or back-up plan in case the alliance fails. The partnership or the project itself may fail. Therefore, it is only good business practice to make sure that there is a back-up plan and strategy defined that could be implemented if necessary.

We have to remember that, in any business dealings, we cannot guarantee the outcomes. The only thing that we can do is ensure that we have done the appropriate research, and done it well, to make the right or best decisions.

If there is a clear understanding of these issues and the conclusion is drawn that an alliance or partnership, in fact, is a viable, acceptable, and the most appropriate approach to take, then, perhaps it is time to go to the dance to meet some potential partners. It is important to keep in mind that this action/approach must be fully supported and accepted by all levels of the organization, especially by the key stakeholders and senior management.

One way to ensure full support and acceptance from all levels of the organization is to ensure that there is a clear evaluation process that the organization will go through to choose the best partner. Along with an accepted and understood process, the criteria for decisions should be well defined and accepted. The process should be effective, efficient, and achievable in a timely manner. In many cases, timing is essential. Taking too much time to do too much at the wrong time can lead to many missed opportunities.

B. Dance With Many Potential Partners

As we all have done at some time in our lives at a dance, we immediately seek out potential partners to whom we are attracted by first impressions. Ask them to dance, but do not stop there. Seek out other potential partners who may not be your first choice. By expanding your potential partner universe, a better choice may become apparent. During the dance, you can talk with the partner, get a feel as to who they are and what they are looking for, or if they are looking for anything at all. It may be that a potential partner who looks "attractive," at first, may not want to talk with you or pursue an alliance.

Once you have danced with many potential partners, take a step back and go through some defined criteria (i.e., items that are specifically important to you) to determine which, with a very preliminary determination, seem like a good match. Some suggested criteria are

- corporate size
- geographic location
- market presence (industry standing, geographic diversity, etc.)
- product portfolio (branded products, generics, innovative products, me-too's, old products, therapeutic value, cost effectiveness, competitive advantages, etc.)
- R&D portfolio (technical innovation, breadth and scope, depth, development stages, etc.)
- R&D technology base (cutting edge or classical, technological partners, scientific credibility, academic associations, etc.)
- therapeutic areas of focus (synergistic with yours, overlapping, expanding, level of expertise, etc.)
- financial stability and profitability
- public or private company
- overall reputation.

Now that you have identified a series of criteria with appropriate gradations and/or definitions of good versus bad, create a prioritized list of the companies, separate them by tiers, where tier one looks like the best match, followed by tier two, and maybe tier three. With a prioritized list, the in-depth search can begin. One of the most common pitfalls in pursuing an alliance is that many companies create a "short-list" of the most likely potential partners very early without appropriate due diligence. The result may be that the best partner is one that is not even considered. On the other hand, there is a danger of overanalysis, which leads to the common problem of "analysis-paralysis." In these cases, analyses/assessments go on forever, and no action is ever taken. This is a very "safe" approach, because an alliance, probably, will never be formed, the company will be busy analyzing and assessing and not doing, and therefore, the risk of a failed alliance will be avoided.

If you have identified a good potential partner, it is possible that the company you have identified may be courting others as well. In these cases, the company that can act quickly, efficiently, effectively, and deliberately will win. There is very little written about the deals that did not happen or the suitors who missed their chance. However, any one involved in the area of alliances and deals has experienced "the one that got away." Because this is a fast moving evolving environment, growth and success are with those who can move expeditiously.

Overall, there needs to be an appropriate balance between effective and thorough analyses and the ability to act quickly. We are living in a very dynamic environment that is changing faster than it ever has. We need to be able to take advantage of and capitalize on opportunities quickly in order to gain and/or maintain a competitive advantage. The balance of complete analysis versus rapid action, however, is different between various companies, and is based on their own internal corporate culture. If any company wishes to change, this is one area that should be addressed first.

C. Learn Everything There is to Know About as Many Partners as You Can

At this point, you should have gotten around the initial infatuation phase and moved on to the assessment of a "real" potential partner. Now, you need to learn everything there is to know about them.

Each potential partner needs to be evaluated objectively. This may be hard to do when members of your organization get stuck on a single potential partner or are reluctant to accept data and/or information counter to their individual perception of the environment. However, objectivity is critical to making good decisions and should be sought. A list of standard criteria with clear definitions and gradations of good versus bad should be used as a framework to build a knowledge base about each potential partner. Many of the same criteria mentioned before could be used again. However, the assessment should be more thorough and in greater detail, with an increase in the depth of information sought.

The criteria defined are those that your organization feels are necessary to determine if there is a good fit/match between the organizations.

This point is easy to define, if you have done a thorough internal assessment, but hard to do, even harder to do well, and often almost impossible to do effectively, in a very subjective and often ill-defined, hidden or guarded environment.

D. Try to Understand Their Goals, Objectives, and Motivation

If you have done a thorough internal assessment, your own goals, objectives and motivations for pursuing an alliance partner have been well defined. It is a challenge to try to put yourself in your potential partner's shoes to understand why they are looking for a partner. It may be helpful to try conducting a parallel evaluation using your own criteria but forming your potential partner's perspectives of themselves. In some cases, reasons for or against a partnership will be very clear. In others, it will not. The key is to try, at least, to list what you feel are their reasons for wanting an alliance with you and then, to determine if any of those reasons could be counterproductive to your own.

For example, if you are looking to learn a new technology to incorporate, eventually, into your own organization and your potential partner is looking for ways to build their own ability and expertise using "their" technology for potential growth as a "service provider," then, they may not be willing to share their technology with you. Therefore, both company's goals and expectations are different. If an alliance is formed under such conditions, there is a good chance that problems will be encountered down the road.

In another case, perhaps you have discovered a new drug that is outside of your core therapeutic areas but would like to grow this area internally. You find a potential partner who is an "expert" in this area to help you develop your new drug. The partner may have other reasons to partner with you, such as filling a hole in their pipeline or the need to pay for internal capacity. In this case, the motivations are different but not necessarily detrimental to either party and, in fact, may be mutually beneficial.

The key is to know, up-front, the reasons both parties want to form an alliance and be willing to accept each other's goals and expectations, even if they are different from yours but not detrimental, obtrusive, or obstructive. Both parties, however, need to be specific and avoid generalities. Without clarity and detail, it is possible that both parties walk away with different interpretations of the "agreed upon goals." If this is the case, then, the opportunities for future problems grow exponentially.

V. COURTSHIP: DO THE ORGANIZATIONS MESH?

Once you have effectively and objectively evaluated the potential partners, it is time to get to know the top choices better. At this point, it is necessary to determine if there is a good cultural, organizational, and philosophical match between the organizations. After all, we are looking for long-term relationships. Therefore, we need to understand and know each other.

Before embarking on an in-depth assessment of potential partners, it is necessary to gauge the level of commitment of your own organization. Is your organization ready, willing, and able to commit time, money, and effort to an alliance for the long term? Once your own internal level of commitment has been firmly established, then, it is time to start looking at potential partners very carefully.

In evaluating each potential partner, it is essential to gain an understanding, to the extent possible, of the level of internal commitment of your potential partner(s) to a possible alliance. If you can find any doubt in the management of either organization that partnering is a good idea, that is good enough reason to look for a different partner or abandon the idea of an alliance, joint venture, or partnership all together.

Most of the work done so far has been at arm's length, focused on internal efforts. Now is the time to make an effort to go out and visit the potential partners to see if they are really interested in working with you. All of these discussions are of a nonconfidential nature to determine levels of interest, corporate synergy, and compatibility of personal chemistry. These areas are not easily quantified, but can be assessed based on

- company history,
- historical growth trends,
- development project mix and R&D strengths,
- marketed product mix and proprietary market position and/or protection (i.e., therapeutic areas, branded, generics, injectables, topicals, OTC, etc.),
- company size (number of people and annual sales),
- company financial situation,
- geographic base (i.e., where is the home office: U.S., Europe, Japan, etc.),
- global presence,
- corporate structure (number of managerial layers, divisional structure, etc.),
- alliance/partnership history and experience, and

- regulatory position (product problems or recalls, FDA inspection results, etc.).

Information on all of these items is generally available from multiple sources. Some can be verified via direct interaction with the potential partners, and all will give you an overall sense of what the company is like, what their problems are, areas of concern, and possible areas of need. In all cases, as was mentioned previously, both parties in any long-term relationship need to feel that they are wanted, needed, trusted, and will benefit from the joint venture/alliance. A clear understanding of each other's needs, goals, and expectations will enhance the ability of both parties to realize how both can benefit from what kind of alliance.

One aspect often given inadequate attention is the issue of geographic and ethnic cultural differences. We are all aware or have heard about the cultural differences associated in dealing with Japanese companies, but do we really understand them, prepare for them, work through them, or do we simply acknowledge them and hope that we can work through them when the time comes?

The Japanese/Western difference is an obvious one, but there are just as many cultural differences between the U.S. and the U.K., or Germany, France, Switzerland, Sweden, Australia, or Canada. One of the most frequently overlooked issues is one of language. From a U.S. perspective, we often feel that if a company speaks "English," we will have no problem in communicating. However, we often forget that we speak "American English" not "British English" or "proper English" which is taught in the local schools. Therefore, many problems are created unknowingly based on a perception that each "understands" the other when both have very different vocabularies and interpretations of the words used.

However, this phenomenon is not unique to companies of different countries. It has also been found between companies of the same country. For example, a discussion between two American companies regarding milestones about a clinical study start and stop could lead to problems. Unknowingly, both companies may have different definitions of these points. For example, to one company, "study start" means when a protocol is signed, to others, when clinical supplies are shipped or when the first patient enters the study, still in others, it is when the first patient actually takes drug. The same kind and number of differences can be seen with definitions of "study stop." Stop can mean when the last patient finishes the study, when all supplies and CRFs are retrieved, when the data base is locked, or when a study report is signed. This is a simple example, which can become very troublesome when progress is reviewed or milestone payments are determined by completion of stated actions.

Other than language and geographically or ethnically defined cultural differences, as described above, there is also the aspect of corporate cultures. Some items to look for and, then, compare to your own corporate culture are listed below. All of these things cannot be quantitatively or objectively quantified. Some of the best ways to get a feel about these things is to talk with the secretaries or visit the company lunchroom, if they have one. Other ways are to talk with executive recruiters, past employees, consultants, their advertising agencies, or meeting people at national or international industry/academic meetings (e.g., PhRMA meetings, American College of Cardiology, BIO-conferences, etc.)

- Formality: Is the company formal or informal, do they have "dress down" days, or is there a generally accepted "uniform"?
- Environment and Atmosphere: Is there a feeling of pressure or anxiety within the company, or does it seem that people are feeling good about what they do, the company and their future? Is the atmosphere quiet and somber or bustling and energetic?
- Bureaucracy: All organizations have formal processes and procedures, but are they rigid or flexible? Are there multiple levels of approval necessary for almost everything, or is responsibility fairly widely distributed?
- Communication Flow and Patterns: Does it appear that communication flows easily up, down, and horizontally, or is there some "unwritten communication protocol" implying that communications between departments or divisions have to go up through the hierarchy in one department or division to the top, the "Chiefs" talk or exchange written correspondence, and then, it goes down into the other department or division? Does it appear that information, both good and bad, flows easily in all directions, or is there a desire to relay only information that confirms or conforms to expectations? Are person-to-person discussions favored over written communications?
- Organizational Structure: An organizational structure can describe or imply how a company will operate.
  ⇒ Is the structure relatively flat, or are there multiple levels with strict reporting lines?
  ⇒ Are there more "Chiefs" (by title) than "Indians"?

$\Rightarrow$ Are they a "centralized" organization or a "decentralized" one? Do they look globally or regionally?

With the comparison of company cultures, if you find differences, the question needs to be asked whether or not these differences are detrimental or could be disruptive to an efficiently functioning alliance. If there is a concern over the ability to work within or through your potential partner's culture (i.e., conflicts or concerns over intercompany or personal chemistry), perhaps it is better to look for another partner.

An additional point that should be addressed here, or earlier, is the need to conduct effective and thorough due diligence of and by both parties. Both should be comfortable with what they have and/or can offer, as well as what the other has and offers. If there is any question in this regard, now is the time to object, not after the contracts are signed. Although, in most cases, every effort is made by both parties to learn all that they can, there is a chance that some things may be overlooked or their importance may not be fully realized. Many of these kinds of things can be, and are, found only after both parties are actively involved in the project itself. Based on this realization, it is important to ensure that mechanisms are put in place to effectively deal with these types of issues. One of the key outcomes of due diligence efforts, from both perspectives, is to assure the partners that the other has what they say they have and can do what they say they can do, when they say they can do it.

VI. MARRIAGE: CONSUMMATION OF THE EVENT

Prior to the actual event, there is a period of engagement, where there is generally a more intimate relationship defined by sharing of confidential information. Unfortunately, at this stage, there are often meetings of the appropriate executives and lawyers, but rarely of the individuals who will actually be involved in the project or work at hand. Therefore, in many cases, contracts are signed and cooperation is defined on paper, with all of the best intentions, but without a real understanding of how it will work in the real world.

Hopefully, at this point there is a mutual agreement as to the overall project, the risks associated with it, its stage of development, and commercial/economic potential. If there is disagreement and/or an unclear picture of any one of these elements or if there is an unrealistic expectation of the potential value or benefit to be gained from participating in the alliance, there will, likely, be a souring of the relationship sooner rather than later, even if a contract is signed. It is unrealistic to assume that economic expectations of either investment or return can be corrected as time progresses. It also must be clearly understood that there is a risk associated with any R&D project and nothing is a guarantee. But the level of risk and the key issues and uncertainties surrounding the project must be clearly defined and understood by all parties before a formal agreement is signed.

With actual contractual execution, certain boundaries are defined, but often levels of detail are not addressed in a formal agreement. Therefore, it is incumbent on the people actually involved with the work, from both organizations, to clearly define for themselves the following areas of activity.

A. Project Specification

What, specifically, is the project that will be carried out? This is not a broad scope definition, but rather a specific and detailed description of the project to be undertaken with definition of

- overall project goal/objective,
- clear definition of what is going to be done and who is going to do it,
- definition of milestones and decision points,
- specification of a schedule,
- specification of overall project costs delineated on either an annual basis for each planned activity in a given year or for expenses projected to reach each identified milestone, and
- clear definition of decision criteria, data required to make those decisions, and studies to provide those data (i.e., what constitutes a good versus a bad outcome, what are the go/no-go criteria, etc.).

B. Operational Processes and Procedures

In general, these are mundane things that most people would not consider too important in the grand scheme of the overall project. However, these simple elements can and do lead to misgivings and bad feelings on both sides. Each of the items listed below really deals with various levels and forms of communication within a respective party of the alliance and between the alliance partners. Each item describes an area that should be part of an overall communication policy/process that both parties understand and adhere to. As in many relationships, problems often result from lack of and/or poor communication. Prospectively addressing these elements can substantially decrease the potential for problems over the long term.

Because these items can easily derail a potentially beneficial partnership, it is prudent to clearly specify joint communication policies, procedures, and processes to deal with the following:

- Define who are the decision makers, how decisions will be made, and how they will be communicated: In most cases, it is advisable to create an Executive Board, composed of equal numbers from both companies, but with a clear mechanism for who has the overall authority to break any deadlocks. This type of forum is essential for major alliance/joint venture issues, but should not be the forum for technical or discipline specific issues, such as clinical, marketing or formulations. These types of issues, problems and questions should be dealt with at technical level committees. In some cases, such as an R&D committee, it is advisable to include Marketing representation to insure commonality of vision and action.
- Define the process for problem resolution: In creating a problem resolution process, it should be emphasized that the earlier a problem is revolved by the lowest possible hierarchical level, the better. In as many cases as possible, the people actually doing the work should resolve the specific problem. For example, the inclusion/exclusion criteria for a clinical protocol should be defined by the clinical experts, as long as the criteria are in line with the overall study objective. In some instances, however, issues and questions arise that could affect more than one area. In these instances, the relevant experts in the appropriate disciplines from both companies must be brought into the decision making process.
- Clarify how information, both good and bad, will be shared and discussed: It must be clearly defined who gets to see what and when. Because both parties should be equally involved in the success of the project, both partners must be intimately involved and privy to all information.
- Report Generation: A procedure needs to be developed that defines who sees and reviews data and, then, who will write individual study reports, how they will be reviewed and approved, and by whom. It is important to include an "expert review" by a panel composed of experts from both companies to review, query, and interpret all data from an experiment or study, agree on the outcome, and then, create a report. If a report is created first, it is much more difficult to change the interpretation or ask more questions. In many cases, defensive positions are taken by authors who may feel that their individual ability as "experts" is being challenged.

- Progress Reporting: The mechanism as to how, when, and by whom progress will be reported needs to be defined. From an R&D perspective, it should be the appointed responsible Project Manager/ Leader with access to all R&D information from all sources in both companies.
- Publication Policy: The publication policy needs to be defined, specifying who writes, reviews, and approves manuscripts, and also when it will be submitted for publication and where.
- Unexpected Findings: A process needs to be defined to explain how to deal with unexpected findings, especially those that may prompt a change in project direction.
- Outside Communication Policy: In an environment of multiple internal and external stakeholders (or stockholders) the activities, progress, and outcomes of organizations become part of the public domain. Therefore, a prospective approach and policy should be developed to generate and disseminate external communications. All inquires from external sources should be funneled through a single source so that only one story is presented to the outside world.

C. Ownership, Responsibility, and Authority

These are always delicate issues within any cooperative alliance. However, as with procedures, they can lead to problems if they are not addressed prospectively. Many of these points will be determined by the project in question and where expertise lies. In all cases, however, because there needs to be a high level of trust and mutual respect between the parties, none of these elements can be completely one-sided.

One other aspect that must be considered is the need to ensure that the key stakeholders in the alliance are actively involved in the operation and definition of the terms and conditions specifying how the alliance will be structured, managed, and monitored. Following up on the point of ensuring that the key stakeholders are actively involved, there should be an alliance "champion" in each partner's organization who will be the internal advocate of the alliance and take every advantage to support and defend it over time.

Along with assuring that the right people are involved at the appropriate time, there are several other issues that should be addressed, such as

- Defining who has the responsibility and will be held accountable for directing, managing, and leading the project. It must be clearly understood that you cannot hold a team or committee accountable.

There must be specific individuals who assume the responsibility and accountability for the success of the partnership/venture. There may be individuals who are assigned the responsibility, accountability and authority for a specific portion of the project, such as R&D, Marketing, Finance, Legal, etc., but there must be a person who assumes overall project responsibility and accountability.

- Defining how problems, conflicts and concerns will be managed and rectified and who will be assigned the responsibility and authority to ensure that they are.
- Clearly defining who owns the data and where it will reside.
- Describing who owns the regulatory submission.
- Defining who is the liaison between the alliance, the regulatory agencies, and the role of each of the partners.
- Defining the managerial structure, specifying that group's responsibility and authority over the various aspects of the alliance's operation. The managerial structure must be straightforward and well understood. The alliance's managerial structure should be developed and geared to ensure the *shared success* of the venture over the long term. In this case, the simpler and clearer the structure, the better. This particular point needs to be tied to and clearly integrated into any discussion about procedures and processes for operating the alliance.

D. Miscellaneous Issues

There are always a few issues and questions that cannot be easily categorized but should not be overlooked. Some of them are

- defining a plan of action for the course to take if the project fails;
- defining how costs will be budgeted, monitored, accounted for, verified, shared or reimbursed, if necessary;
- specifying, to the degree of certainty possible, if there will need to be an additional investment over the current R&D budget by entering into the alliance and/or how current R&D budgets will be allocated to the alliance project;
- defining, up-front, where the money will come from, both partners or one.

E. Project Team Structure, Management, and Operation

One of the key aspects in defining how an alliance will work is defining how the project will be managed. In most cases, a team is created to oversee the project and ensure that it keeps moving forward. Although formation of a team seems to be certain in almost every situation, there are some basic concepts and issues that should not be overlooked.

Overall, formation of a team to manage a joint venture/alliance R&D project encompasses its own nuances that may make it different from the teams that either partner normally creates to manage internal projects. Some basic questions to ask are

- What kind of team will be created to manage the project (i.e., technical specialist team, development team, integrated interdisciplinary team, R&D/marketing team, etc.)?
- Who will participate in the team (i.e., equal representation from both partners, only one company, overall size of the team, etc.)?
- Who will lead the team (i.e., Project Manager, Project Leader, or Project Director from which company)?
- What will be the responsibility and authority of the team and the team leader (i.e., who establishes, enforces, and reinforces)?
- How will the team operate (i.e., logistics, such as, where, when, frequency, etc.)?

Selecting the team leader, with the appropriate hierarchical level, ability, knowledge, and personal interactive skills is a difficult challenge even for internal projects. A joint venture/alliance project is even more difficult. The individual has to be accepted by both organizations and viewed as an individual who can effectively work through and with potentially diverse groups of people with different motivations and agendas. Some factors that can enhance the project leader's effectiveness are

- the alliance project should be the only responsibility;
- no affiliation with any local/internal project team associated with the alliance project;
- a physical and organizational position which is viewed as an objective "outsider."

Implementing these few factors sends a strong message to both organizations. Overall, it will be perceived that both organizations feel that this project is important enough that these bold steps have been taken, and also it provides an opportunity for the project leader to assume full-time ownership of the alliance project and help assure its success.

However, appointing a project leader is only the first step down the road to a successful relationship. The project leader has to take a position of objectivity, but from a different perspective. This individual should

- focus on the global project and organizational issues, not daily concerns or actions; and
- maintain very close association with the key departments and individuals who have the greatest impact on the overall success of the project.

From a functional perspective, the project leader should not be the one doing the work, but rather the individual who removes the "roadblocks" and "greases the skids" to let the technical experts get the job(s) done. Secondly, the project leader should ensure that what is being done is part of the overall project plan (i.e., ensure that the "right" tasks are identified, and then work to ensure that the path is clear to get them done well, on time, and within budget). Taking this perspective forces the project leader to use clairvoyant and intuitive powers to prospectively look forward and anticipate where and when problems may occur and take steps to eliminate and/or minimize those factors before they can influence project progress.

As we all know, no matter how effective a project leader is, problems will occur. It is advisable, however, to work through the problems rather than taking them "up to management" for resolution. Overall, it is beneficial to find solutions through the teams and technical experts and not push the problem up the hierarchy. Also, the project leader needs to take the position of not solving the problems for the team members, but rather encouraging them to solve the problems. In all instances, it is important to keep the management of both organizations informed of what is happening, but the project leader should take the perspective that they are informing and, perhaps, seeking advice, but not searching for answers or solutions. Taking this approach with both the team and management reinforces the concept of team empowerment and enhances the project leader's effectiveness as a leader and facilitator.

This is not to say that the project leader should be a "wallflower" but must keep a global/big-picture focus on the project. The project leader should challenge individuals and team actions and approaches, for the sake of global outcomes but should not challenge details and technical matters; these issues and questions can be raised directly by and/or through a technical expert.

Overall, it is very important for the project leader to be visible. There is no substitute for face-to-face contact and established personal rapport. Therefore, the project leader should be at both sites equally.

The team should be the venue for making project-related decisions. Therefore, once a decision is made, there should be no reason to revisit it unless it is absolutely necessary. From this perspective, the alliance project team should be in harmony as to what needs to be done, who is going to do it, and when it will be done.

The alliance project leader, however, can be set up to fail, either intentionally or unintentionally. Both partners have to accept the role and responsibility of the project leader with freedom to do the job. If the following are not defined or accepted by both organizations for the project leader, the team and team leader will have little chance to succeed:

- a role that is well defined and clearly communicated;
- defined scope of responsibility, authority and accountability, accepted or reinforced (i.e., when ever a problem arises that is brought to line management, the line manager redirects the problem to the project leader rather than solving it themselves);
- well-defined decision making responsibility; and
- clear mechanism for budgetary control and/or direct influence.

Overall, the success of a project leader depends on the ability to influence, which depends on credibility and trust built on mutual respect.

The team structure/membership is always a challenge, especially with an alliance partner. In many cases, in an attempt not to offend anyone, teams become inordinately large, with duplicate experts from both organizations as members. In itself, this is a dysfunctional team. It is always beneficial to keep teams small. Therefore, from an overall project management perspective, an alliance project team structure can be viewed as multiple teams, governed by a common "core team," headed by the project leader. The core team should include a clinical leader, a nonclinical leader with responsibility for all nonclinical functions, a regulatory affairs leader, local project managers (if they exist), and a marketing leader. Manufacturing representation should be added at the appropriate time within a project's development life cycle. As is the case with many of the nonclinical functions, their level of input and/or their required input waxes and wanes over the time course of the project. In some cases and at some times, manufacturing and some of the nonclinical functional areas can be viewed as "agenda team members" whose representation is required for a specific agenda topic or part of a project's development. In any case, it is imperative to ensure that the right people are available at the right time to give the best input.

Each of the core team members then leads a technical area specific team, which has input to the core team through its leaders or core team agenda members, as appropriate. The overall scheme of the core team and its affiliate teams is described in Fig. 1.

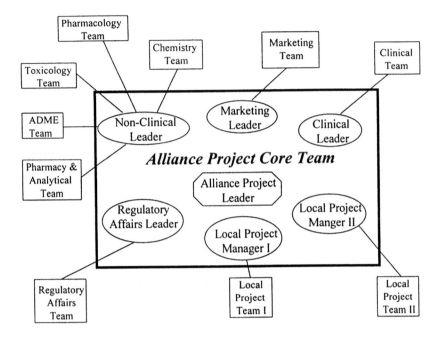

FIG. 1 Alliance project core team concept.

VII. THE HONEYMOON AND LEARNING TO LIVE TOGETHER: THE PERIOD OF EUPHORIA AND POSSIBLE DISILLUSIONMENT

The honeymoon is a period when the planning and definition of all working aspects of the alliance are tested in a real situation. This is when the partners realize that their expectations were correct, or they were not.

In almost every case, there will be bumps and grinds as the processes and procedures start to be implemented. There is also a customary learning phase when productivity declines in favor of bringing both parties up to speed on the project, its history, and fine details of each other's organization.

This is also a period when not much really gets done. There is a lot of discussion and contemplation on how and when to do what was defined previously. During this time, there is either the realization that what the "owner" of the project thought was "right" is confirmed by the partner, or the opposite occurs. In the first case, there is a real state of optimism and euphoria. If the opposite scenario occurs, there is a feeling of disillusionment and concern.

Overall, both scenarios are generally short-lived and may not be the entire picture. One would hope that appropriate due diligence was exerted by both parties prior to consummation of the deal, but it is not uncommon to uncover certain facts or surprises when the actual work gets started.

Also, during this time, both partners generally experience mixed emotions. The company that originated the idea or technology may start having feelings of incompetence. This is often due to the perception that "we could not do it ourselves," or "we couldn't do it right," or "our management did not have enough faith in us to think that we could do it right at a reasonable cost and on time." Therefore, a partner had to be found. In addition, the partner may adapt the feeling of "NIH: Not Invented Here" syndrome, where there is rejection of the idea or it is relegated to a low-priority position in the general scheme of work on a personal level. Partners may also take a position of perceived superiority assuming the same reasons the originator did and believing they are the "white knight" to save the project from ruin. All of these ideas and perceptions will exist to some degree in both organizations. In entering this phase of the partnership, these points must be understood, and effectively addressed early.

A lot of the good, bad, and the ugly will appear during this time. However, it also has to be understood that this period forms the basis of a long-term relationship and that the overall success of the alliance can be significantly affected, positively or negatively, during this time. If the euphoria, concerns, and/or problems can be dealt with proactively, quickly, efficiently, and with a spirit of cooperation, a positive basis for the future of the alliance can be built. If the opposite occurs, either real or imagined, the seeds are sown for a rocky relationship.

After the honeymoon, the alliance moves into a phase when both parties should be actively involved in the project. This is also when both parties are still getting to know each other, learning to work within their partner's company culture and operations, and trying to make progress in the project. During this time, all of the procedures, practices, and processes that were defined up-front are tested. As with any new venture, when new activities are implemented, there will be times when they obviously do not work and must be revised and new ideas will be proposed. Modifications must be made, some procedures must be changed, others deleted, and, at other times, new ones must be developed, based on the evolving environment of the new alliance. A word of caution must be interjected here. It is always easy to criticize a given procedure. However, before established alliance procedures are disregarded or changed, they should be tried. In many cases, evolution will be a much better approach than revolution. The acceptance of the changes and they way they are handled by the management of both partners and the alliance will demonstrate how committed both are to the partnership. Organizations are very astute, and they form perceptions and/or draw conclusions from what they see, hear, or assume. As is always the case, perception becomes reality, even if it is wrong. During these times, the necessity of clear and concise communication channels can not be overemphasized. Even if actions occur or do not occur, as long as there is a reasonable explanation, most people will accept the outcome.

We also have to keep in mind that, in most cases, this is an unsettling time for many. We are asking both parties to change and learn to live and work differently than they did before. Change is a very frightening thing for many people. Initiating a partnership with an outside company can be seen as threatening to some and invigorating or exciting to others. All possibilities along the continuum of acceptance to outright rejection will probably be seen among the players involved with the project from both companies. Successful alliances can effectively deal with this level of concern or resistance to change. If it is ignored, another seed of failure is planted.

This is a period of learning, experimenting, and gaining a sense if both parties are actively committed to making the partnership work. At this stage of the partnership, neither party can become placid or ignore the reality of people's perceptions and concerns. In these instances, the management team of both companies can "never fail to lead." Every action will be watched and dissected. Seemingly unrelated events and actions will be coupled, and erroneous conclusions and perceptions will be drawn. Failure to realize that this is a normal and real part of any organizational change will plant another seed for future problems.

VIII. MATURITY AND STABILIZATION: MAKING IT WORK FOR THE DURATION

There are several factors that come into play over the long term for maintaining alliances. Some appear to be common sense, like communication channels. Others are not so clear. Unfortunately, many of the common sense things are often overlooked, resulting in problems that could have been easily avoided. Following are some of the key points to watch.

A. Communication

For the long haul, the most important factor is developing and fostering multiple and open communication channels. Communication needs to flow up, down, and across, clearly and unencumbered. The more filters in place, the lower the chance that a true picture will emerge. Problems will occur within the alliance. The successful alliances will see and act on those concerns before they become divisive perceptions.

B. Long-Term Commitment

As time passes in any relationship, it is easy to become passive and begin to take things for granted. It is easy to assume that things will continue as they have been, and therefore, the amount of attention paid to the partner and/or the alliance diminishes. If a perception is created that one partner is taking the other for granted or no longer cares, it is very easy for the alliance overall to deteriorate.

When dealing with organizations or in any personal relationship, it takes a lot less energy to maintain a positive environment than it does to reverse a negative situation or perception. If there is a reduction in the amount of energy, effort, or commitment to any relationship, either perceived or real, negative consequences are probable. Therefore, it is advisable to maintain an appropriate level of enthusiasm and commitment to ensure that the alliance continues on a positive trend, rather than spend an excessive amount of time and effort turning around a negative perception or loss of motivation.

In many cases, one of the easiest ways to keep the alliance project in the forefront is to tie its success and progress to individuals' performance assessment. If the work is directly tied to an overall performance assessment, it is unlikely to be forgotten or overlooked. This approach applies to both the workers and the management staff. Managers must also feel that their attention and performance rank are directly tied to the timely progress of the alliance's project.

Both parties should clearly understand, hopefully, before the alliance is consummated, that both partners will have to commit a lot of time and effort continually to insure the long-term success of the alliance. Success of alliance projects does not just happen, it is achieved by patience and commitment.

C. Growth and Evolution: An Awareness of the Environment

Over time, both companies will change, mature, and grow. The external environment is also evolving and changing, often in unexpected directions. The alliance partners need to monitor these internal and external changes, see how they affect the partnership, and adjust accordingly. There is value in stability and consistency. However, there are clear instances when consistency (i.e., not being flexible and/or adapting to environmental changes) is not the appropriate course.

Successful alliances will adapt to a new environment. They will look for ways to enhance the value of the partnership, if it is in their best interest. This is where keen knowledge of your own company and your partner's becomes critical in being able to evolve or become stagnant.

Annual or semiannual reviews of the alliance project, as an entity in itself and as it relates to other internal projects and the external environment, can and do offer opportunities to make modifications or, if necessary, abandon the alliance in favor of an alternative approach or other projects. In any review, however, there must be effective reality checks built into the process. Change in direction for the sake of change is not productive. R&D projects generally have long time frames associated with them. Frequent changes in focus or project priority often lead to frustration and abandonment of the concept and positive initiative that was part of the alliance at the beginning.

D. Project Priority Shift

As in many marriages, passion dissipates with time. The challenge to the alliance management team is to maintain the level of enthusiasm, commitment, and motivation, present at the beginning of the project, over the longterm. Along with frequent changes in focus and/or direction of the project, the other factor that can reduce any level of commitment is a downward shift in the priority of the alliance's project.

In most organizations, a downward shift in priority results in less commitment, less resources, and, more than likely, a delayed time line. This priority shift also sends negative messages throughout both organizations which, if intentional, are very effective and, if not, can be equally devastating. There may be very good reasons for a change in the priority of an alliance project within either partner. However, the change and the reasons for the change need to be clearly conveyed to both parties. In either case, the effect will probably be negative.

Also, it is next to impossible to have a change in priority within one organization without having it become public knowledge in the other. By this time, hopefully, good communication patterns have been established among the people doing the work. If there is a change, that information will be discussed, if for nothing else, to explain why certain resources are not available or why a study is taking longer to complete than anticipated. If changes in priority are kept quiet, the alliance is dealt a major blow to its trust, openness, and respect for the other party.

On the other hand, an upward shift in priority can rejuvenate a stagnating effort or pump new enthusiasm into a project that has lost a bit of its luster over time. This may very well result from the positive outcome of a given study or a positive change in environmental conditions. In any event, such a change will increase interest and motivation among all parties concerned.

E. Openness and Dependence

As time passes, your partner has had an opportunity to learn all there is to know about you. If the relationship is growing and prospering, your partner has learned how to work with you and accept all of your faults and idiosyncrasies. In addition, you have done the same with your partner. If the alliance cooperation level seems to be fading, perhaps, there are specific internal corporate quirks in either company that simply irritate the other partner. If the alliance is to develop and prosper, a mechanism must be defined and used to address these issues.

During the course of any relationship, many, if not all, of your secrets will become known by your partner. In an alliance setting, there is a good possibility that all of your strengths and weaknesses will become obvious to your partner, and theirs to you. In many cases, this is an opportunity to learn and grow but, in some cases, can be seen as a threat. On the positive side, we all know that no one has the market cornered on ideas. Under that philosophy, an alliance provides each partner with an opportunity to learn from each other and adopt practices, procedures, or approaches to enhance your own ability to develop competitive advantages or organizational efficiencies. On the negative side, your current competitive advantages may become known by your partner, and therefore, could no longer be considered an advantage.

Partnerships require an open and free environment to succeed. However, in most cases, alliances and joint ventures are related to specific projects or products. Internal operations that provide you with a unique information source or market assessment do not necessarily have to be brought into the alliance, unless they are specific to the project or product in question. Either partner can keep parts of their business operations to themselves and/or only provide an output or service to the alliance. In this way, some corporate attributes or secrets can still remain confidential.

Overall, it is important to address these issues. Many of them will not become obvious until the project is moving along and the partners are working closely together. It does help, however, to generally understand what you feel are the "family jewels" worth protecting and what can be shared with a partner throughout an alliance.

There is a possibility, through this close level of cooperation, that either partner may start to consider itself or be considered an integral part of the other. Also, either party may feel that its identity is now defined as the "alliance/partnership" not as independent organizations cooperating on a project.

In such a case, either partner may become a core element in the other's overall business strategy and an integral part of the other's business. This may be bad or good. It is good, if this is realized, accepted, and endorsed by both parties. It could be bad because one of the partners may realize this and the other does not, or, as time passes, one acquires the other. In such a case, the one partner simply ceases to exist and is totally incorporated into the other partner. This often happens when one partner is significantly larger, such as when a large pharmaceutical company forms an alliance with a small biotechnology or biomedical company. In the beginning, the larger company has a need that is fulfilled by the smaller company. If the larger company determines over time that this "technology or service" is vital to its future operations or competitive ability, it may simply acquire the smaller company. This, in fact, is a common long-term strategy of many smaller biotechnology/biomedical companies (i.e., to be acquired).

This is not necessarily bad, especially if the smaller company fully supports and agrees to the acquisition. It could be detrimental if the opposite is true. In such a case, the ability, technology, or service that the larger company wanted or needed, may become only part of the larger company on paper. The intellectual capacity to perform (i.e., the people with the expertise, knowledge and ability), may simply leave the organization. If this occurs, then, the larger company acquired a hollow shell and will probably never fully realize the outcome they hoped to gain through the acquisition.

IX. AMIABLE SEPARATION OR MESSY DIVORCE: WERE GOALS REALIZED OR WERE PROMISES/EXPECTATIONS BROKEN?

As time passes and more information is available from internal and external sources, it may become obvious to either one or both parties that dissolution of the alliance is necessary, or it may be beneficial to the economic health of either or both parties. Separation is not necessarily bad. If separation is for positive reasons and both parties agree, the separation, in fact, can be amiable and beneficial.

Obviously there are many reasons for dissolving a partnership, both positive and negative. It must also be clear that it is unwise to maintain a partnership when, clearly, it should be dissolved. In these cases, several arguments are raised for continuing the partnership, such as the amount of time, energy, and money invested so far (The concept of "sunk cost" can not be supported as a valid reason for continuing an alliance when there is clear reason for dissolution, but it is used.), reluctance to realize that the situation needs to change, or a selfish reason (either personal or corporate). In all of these examples, the pain of dissolution is not as bad as the damage possible from continuing. One always has to determine if it is better to live in misery or under guarded conditions in the hope of salvaging something at the end or to break the relationship cleanly and move on.

If there are negative reasons for breaking the alliance, such as deterioration of trust, respect, or communication, there are opportunities to revive the partnership with the help of a mediator, a consultant, or a more active role of the alliance's managerial staff. However, both parties must feel that there is something worth saving and are willing to put in the effort to make it work. In some cases, the effort needed may be more than one or both parties are willing to expend. In other cases, the real reason for the separation may not be one that people really want to hear. In either case, clean separation is better than the lingering misery of continued cohabitation.

During the course of an alliance, there can be many valid reasons presented for dissolving the partnership. As in any long-term relationship, arguments will erupt and differences of opinion can create walls, hostility, and communication barriers. In a strong alliance, avenues are available to deal with differences and problems, and resolution is straightforward and fair. However, if the means to resolve problems are not well defined or procedures are in place that simply do not work or are not used, separations can and do occur for the wrong reasons.

Relationships have soured because of unrealistic expectations of what the alliance can do, is willing to provide, or will deliver in either product/ project, information, or economic terms. In either case, these types of reasons for messy divorces are mainly the result of insufficient preparation and investigation before the deal is consummated. This factor is one that can be either internal or external. Therefore, as mentioned previously, a complete internal assessment and an evaluation of the potential partner must be done and done well to avoid future pitfalls.

Of course, there are clear success stories as well, where everything goes as expected and true outcomes are realized. In some cases, there are defined outcomes over a certain period of time as measures of the success. In other cases, there are different measures of success for each respective partner. If the goals and critical success factors are synergistic, or, at least, not detrimental to the other party, it is much easier for both companies and the alliance to succeed. The experience that companies have in dealing with partners varies and has an impact on the potential success of future alliances. Therefore, if your particular company has been involved with many alliances, there is a greater likelihood that future partnerships will succeed. Based on actual hands-on experience, you know the types of things to look out for, the things to do up-front, and the kinds of partnerships to develop.

Likewise, companies that have had bad experiences with alliances of any sort will probably tend to shy away from them in the future or create a situation that is so one-sided that a partner never really feels like a "partner," but rather as an associate or a contractor. In either of these cases, a large part of the potential benefit that could be gained from an alliance is often lost.

First time players in the alliance/partnership game can be viewed as being either at an advantage or disadvantage. Because of their lack of pertinent hands-on experience, they may overlook some of the basic elements necessary for building successful alliances, or they may be fortunate enough to pair up with a company with a positive history of partnerships that can help guide the way. The disadvantages are obvious. Liberties can be taken by the partner and unfair terms and conditions can be stipulated, all of which can detract from the potential value that could be gained from an alliance.

We have to remember that an alliance should have an outcome greater than the sum of the individual players. Both partners need to feel trusted, respected, and comfortable that they are or have benefited from the time and effort spent in the alliance. If not, perhaps one or both did not bring their full commitment, trust, respect, enthusiasm, and motivation into the alliance from the beginning.

X. SUMMARY AND CONCLUSIONS

Effective and productive alliances, joint ventures, and partnerships, like long-term personal relationships, are possible, but not without effort, forethought, thoroughness, patience, commitment, and the desire to make them work.

7

Managing Contracted Clinical Research and Development

The View from the Client and Contract Research Organization

Frank R. Mangan

F.R.M. Associates Consulting Services
Surrey, England

Albert J. Siemens

ClinTrials Research, Inc.
Research Triangle Park, North Carolina

I. RATIONALE FOR CONTRACTING STUDIES TO CONTRACT RESEARCH ORGANIZATIONS (CROs)

In the last ten years, the CRO industry has changed dramatically. During the 80s, pharmaceutical companies used CROs, primarily, as a last resort to implement studies or selected portions thereof, which had been fully planned and organized by the sponsor. Often, the studies were not pivotal. The services contracted could be restricted to selecting and/or initiating study sites, clinical monitoring, or, perhaps, checking case report forms, entering data, or writing a report. The CRO was seen as the agency you turned to when the pharmaceutical company no longer had internal capacity or could not cope with competing requirements, and were very much a last resort providing a short-term solution. In fact, many CROs came into existence through this type of approach by the pharmaceutical industry specializing in data management or clinical monitoring by the very nature of the experience and expertise of their founders [1].

Cost containment measures brought about by health care reforms in the U.S.A. and Europe have resulted in major restructuring within the pharmaceutical industry as executives have responded to the challenges of maintaining the high profits enjoyed throughout the 80s. Many senior pharmaceutical executives are recognizing the synergy which can exist between their company and the CRO industry. Following mergers and acquisitions, downsizing has been very attractive but, in many cases, has led to staff insufficient to cope with the workload. Using a CRO can help a pharmaceutical company manage peaks and troughs in the development cycle without adding more people to the payroll. The next logical step is to consider outsourcing as part of strategic planning, moving the responsibility and risks of hiring, housing, and supporting staff from the pharmaceutical company to the CRO. Consequently, the large fixed costs of clinical development can, then, be managed as variable costs allowing pharmaceutical executives to direct the fixed costs elsewhere, such as to discovery, manufacture, or marketing.

The CRO industry has responded to the changing environment with enormous appetite and with a great deal of success. Individual companies have experienced and continue to experience rapid growth. The industry is currently growing in turnover at a rate of 20–25 percent per annum, and some of the more successful companies are enjoying growth of 40 percent. This growth rate has not been even across all sectors. Those experiencing the highest rate are in clinical monitoring, data management, regulatory affairs, and postmarketing surveillance, whereas Phase I activities have seen only a 5 percent growth [2]. Sponsors are now demanding more comprehensive cover for clinical monitoring, across Europe and particularly in the countries of the former eastern block, and great interest is being expressed about conducting more trials in South America and Australasia. It is now essential that a CRO provides data management and statistical and regulatory services, particularly if they wish to be selected for the potentially lucrative full service contracts. The appearance of drug packaging and labeling facilities within CROs is now also being seen by some clients as a major requirement.

As CROs have become more sophisticated and pharmaceutical companies have undergone major restructuring, the major CROs are increasingly being expected to take key roles in the design, conduct, and full reporting of entire development programs. This applies particularly to Japanese pharmaceutical companies and to the biotechnology industry. The American and European subsidiaries of Japanese companies depend heavily on CROs because they have only recently started to run large scale projects in the West and have not had time to build up the infrastructure required. Most biotechnology companies have a small number of compounds under development and cannot afford to build and maintain the clinical and regulatory departments needed to develop their drugs successfully. However, the requests for involvement at the design stages and full management of programs is not restricted to these two sets of clients. Some major American and European sponsors are also making such requests, often via strategic alliances or preferred supplier agreements [1].

The challenge to the CRO industry through the remainder of the 90s and into the next century is to manage growth without becoming uncompetitive and to continue demonstrating that it can deliver a first-class quality product at a cost to its clients which they cannot match themselves. The challenge is to build and maintain a competitive infrastructure while maintaining profitability. To provide the range and spread of services now required by sponsors demands capital and also a guaranteed cash flow. Many of the major CROs are now public companies, which, although this provides capital for expansion, also brings a need for profitability. Now, they need investor relations departments, advertising, marketing and business development groups, and strong internal administrative departments, such as training, financial accounting, and human resources. There may be an optimal size for a service company like a CRO above which the needs of infrastructure and profit may start to negate potential savings. The medium-sized CRO of today may continue to grow until it, too, reaches optimal size, and the specialist or niche player will likely continue to thrive.

II. ESSENTIAL STEPS TO BE TAKEN WITHIN A PHARMACEUTICAL COMPANY WHEN DECIDING TO CONTRACT OUT STUDIES

From the discussion in the introduction to this chapter, it is clear that the decision to contract out work can be prompted by several reasons. Lack of capacity within the pharmaceutical company used to be the main reason, but now it is becoming increasingly more common for studies to be contracted as a result of a strategic decision. This is particularly so for biotechnology companies, but, in many pharmaceutical companies, a decision has been made to contract out a fixed proportion, perhaps, 20 percent of studies. Whatever the reason for contracting, there are several basic steps which must be followed to allow a smooth flow for the anticipated study. These steps relate to determining budget availability, authorizing the expenditure, responsibilities to be retained and contracted, decision making ability, and responsibility and management of the contract.

The financial aspects of clinical studies have increasingly become the focus of senior management of pharmaceutical companies within the past few years. The total R&D budget of sponsor companies, which has risen by a compound growth rate of 12 percent annually since 1989, has been currently estimated at about $37 billion. For individual companies, the clinical budget is a large proportion of the entire operating budget and is incurred at a strategic stage in the drug development cycle; make a blunder at this stage and all the preclinical work will have been for nothing. Thus, budget setting and managing the clinical budget of a pharmaceutical company has become a very important and increasingly sophisticated activity. Studies must be identified early in plans and costs budgeted, expenditure monitored and accruals made correctly for expenses incurred but not yet invoiced. Many of the larger pharmaceutical companies have established contract departments whose responsibilities include ensuring that studies to be contracted are identified early so that the costs which will be incurred are correctly identified and budgeted.

Some process must be in place to assure that the decision to contract out a study is taken by the appropriate member of staff within an organization and that the decision and the financial implications are communicated to the financial and project management departments. The costs of clinical studies are such that great care should be given to financial authorization levels of those staff members who will contract out studies. A clear authorization process with strict limits should be in place to allow rapid and proper approval of the expenditure.

Once approval to contract has been granted, the first step is to draw up a "Responsibility Checklist." This lists all of the activities in detail which the sponsor wishes to retain and those for which the CRO will be responsible. This is a vital document which forms the basis of discussions with prospective CROs and the basis for the final contract. It is vital that this be completed by each group affected within the sponsor company. The list should start with all those activities needed to prepare for a study, including study design, protocol preparation, CRF design, investigator brochure production, etc., through to sections on study management, study initiation, study conduct, data analysis, and reporting. All aspects of the study must be covered to avoid misunderstanding and confusion of responsibilities, at a later date, between the CRO and sponsor.

It is essential that the Responsibility Checklist be fully communicated throughout the sponsor company and agreed to by each group within the company. The Data Management department must be aware and involved if a study is to be contracted out even if they will not be conducting the analysis themselves. They must agree to the specifications of the data base to be used by the CRO and other aspects. Similarly, the clinical team members must be aware and involved if the analysis of a study is to be contracted out. In fact, the formation of a project team with representatives from each of the functions to agree on the Responsibility Checklist and to agree to the choice of CRO is recommended. In those companies which have chosen to form contracts departments, it is the responsibility of those staff members to ensure that such a team is formed and that decisions taken are communicated effectively throughout the company.

Timings required by the sponsor must be agreed to internally before being communicated to CROs. The team approach mentioned is, again, suggested to facilitate agreement. The timings agreed upon must be achievable and realistic. It is not uncommon to hear a pharmaceutical company staff admit that the timings they require from CROs could not possibly be met internally.

Allocation of responsibility within the pharmaceutical company for decisions to be taken and for the subsequent management of the contract is vital. Although the contract staff may be responsible for ensuring communication of decisions, it must be the project head and budget holder who has decision making authority. Once the study is awarded, it must be clear who within the company is responsible for what. The clinical team or data management team have clear responsibility to oversee the contract and ensure that timings, quality, and patient enrollment are being met. However, it is usually good practice to appoint a contract person for all queries which arise. This avoids confusion and also avoids the possibility that decisions made by one group or person within the company are not communicated to others who may be affected by the decisions. By ensuring that the steps described above are addressed a pharmaceutical company should, at least, start out in control of the contracting process.

III. APPROACHES TO SELECTING A CRO

The CRO market has seen a plethora of mergers and acquisitions in the 90s. In the main, these have been aggressive mergers with the objective of expanding either services offered or widening the geographical cover. Now, the major CROs all offer full service and some, notably Covance, Quintiles, and ClinTrials Research, offer preclinical and clinical services. The major players in these acquisitions have been companies based in the U.S.A. They have acquired operating groups in many European countries and beyond as a response to requests from their major sponsors to conduct global studies. The medium-sized, independent CROs, which have not been acquired, in some cases, have sought to form alliances with others to offer pan-European capabilities or have sought U.S.A.-based partners with whom to work in multinational studies. However, the difficulty of organizing trials to essentially the same standards across several independent organizations has usually proven to be too great a challenge. The joint venture, where all partners have a financial interest in the contracts each other is bidding for, has been much more successful.

Technomark Consulting Services has stated that there are 262 CROs in Europe alone and that there are now eighteen public CROs in the U.S.A. with an equity value approaching $1 billion employing 10,000 staff. Thus, the selection of a CRO is a daunting process for a pharmaceutical, biotechnology, or medical devices company. Technomark Consulting Services produces a register of CROs listing major facilities, senior staff, and a brief description of the services offered which may be a starting point for companies searching for a CRO. However, the register gives no indication of quality of the service offered.

In many pharmaceutical companies, there is little strategy behind choosing a CRO. CROs are used sparingly and the amount contracted varies considerably from year to year. Under these conditions, if a particular CRO has been used before, for example, by the cardiovascular team and has performed a study adequately, then, it will be used again for a similar study in that therapeutic area. Traditionally, a small number of CROs will be used, probably consisting of small, niche, and full service CROs. The decisions to use the CROs will be made by individuals within the company based on personal experience which is commonly limited. This approach can lead to disappointment and dissatisfaction if the CRO has staff changes or is unable to complete the study and can lead to panic and another round of internal information gathering. Often, there has been no attempt to establish a database of experience, and consequently, no coordination is possible when choosing CROs for further studies. This strategy or lack of strategy ensures that many of the benefits of the expertise and scale of performance of CROs are overlooked by the pharmaceutical company. This strategy, thus, penalizes the pharmaceutical company because it will have limited knowledge of CRO costs and performance and will use only the few CROs it works with on a limited number of occasions.

A better approach is to determine that a certain proportion of clinical work will be contracted each year and for the company to make a rigorous selection of CROs with whom they will place contracts. The selection is usually made by a team led by the contracts staff in companies which have established such a group or by a Task Force charged with conducting the project. The first task in such an approach is to determine what the business needs are for the particular pharmaceutical company. The business needs are driven by the following generic factors:

a] are you intending to contract out full service contracts?
b] are you going to contract out international studies and if so across which countries?
c] are you contracting out clinical activities and/or data management and biometrics?

d] do you need specific therapeutic experience?

e] do you have specific needs for database software?

By an examination and agreement on these factors, it should be possible to narrow the number of CROs who offer the services required by your business needs and, thus, reduce the burden of evaluation.

The most common way to start evaluating CROs is to devise a questionnaire. This must be done with great care and thought. Too often, these questionnaires ask for excessive information, much of which is irrelevant to the decision making process. The main questions can be clustered under the following headings:

a) details of company ownership and business history

b) company structure, permanent staff numbers at each site and the distribution across disciplines

c) specific trial experience in the areas to be contracted, including details of countries worked in during the last three years, number of studies, number of sites, and number of patients completed

d) SOPs currently in use internationally and how international conformity with SOPs is achieved and maintained

e) details of project management structure, software, and how international trials are managed

f) CVs (anonymous) of potential Project Managers.

g) description of data management and statistical analytical procedures and how these are effected for international projects

h) description of proposed study requirements and schedule and how they will be met

i) software in common use for trial management, data capture, statistical analysis and word processing.

Information should also be requested on financial matters including access to the last three years' accounts.

The questionnaires need be sent only to those CROs which are expected to meet the company's business needs as agreed beforehand. Knowing which CROs can meet those needs demands considerable knowledge of the industry and, unless the company has an established contracts group, it is probably worthwhile to contact a consultant with the knowledge to help in the selection. Following receipt of the questionnaires completed by the targeted CROs, some can be excluded from further consideration.

The next stage involves site visits to conduct audits of the CRO facilities, policies, and procedures. This may seem unnecessary to some but, in fact, it is vitally important. The company staff who conduct the audits must be chosen with great care. They must be discipline-specific to include all areas to be contracted and also include a financially qualified member. Moreover, the team must devote sufficient time to the task and understand the importance of the visit. The sponsor must set the agenda, and forewarn the CRO of documentation desired, e.g., certificates, SOPs, CVs, etc. Access must be requested to all personnel at all levels and to all facilities, and more than one office of the CRO should be visited if possible.

Failings of the CROs should be reported back to them if it is decided not to include them in the list of CRO candidates.

Then, contracting is concentrated on a carefully selected small number of CROs which can deliver the services required. It should be possible to negotiate so-called "umbrella" contracts to cover all of the major contractual issues leaving the details of specific studies to be added as addenda.

The next logical stage in the CRO–pharmaceutical company arrangement is the preferred partnership into which several major companies have entered recently. This will be discussed in detail in Section IV.

The discussion above has dealt largely with pharmaceutical companies which have already contracted out clinical research and have staff experienced in selecting a CRO and negotiating contracts. However, there are a number of companies which have never contracted studies and have no experienced staff. When they are faced with contracting out a series of studies or even one study, they have a difficult time ahead. However, if they follow the steps outlined above it will make their selection process less prone to error. They can also turn to a number of independent consultants to help them through the stages of selection, negotiation, and management of contracts.

IV. PREFERRED PARTNERSHIPS

In the U.K., a nonprofit company, Partnership Sourcing Ltd., has been set up by the Confederation of British Industry (CBI) and the Department of Trade and Industry (DTI) to increase awareness, knowledge, and the implementation of sourcing partnerships among British companies. A survey conducted by this company of over three hundred companies from all sectors of industry and commerce, including both manufacturing and service sectors, revealed the success of introducing preferred partnerships. Of those companies forming such partnerships, 81 percent were able to improve the service they gave to their customers, 85 percent were able to reduce costs, 78 percent to improve their product quality, and 67 percent to improve delivery times.

The CRO industry provides a service to pharmaceutical companies and is expected by their clients to address those very issues said to be improved in the survey cited of companies in other industries which have introduced preferred partnerships. There is, therefore, a good case for considering such partnerships between a pharmaceutical company and a number of selected and evaluated CROs.

The benefits to the CRO which are central to the formation of preferred partnerships with a number of clients are	The benefits sought by a pharmaceutical company from a preferred partner are
1. to obtain a secure cash flow 2. to reduce the administrative burden of bidding and negotiation for contracts awarded elsewhere 3. to improve forward planning, work scheduling, staff allocation, and recruitment 4. to reduce advertising and business development costs 5. to enhance staff job satisfaction by being part of a team with the client	1. predictable prices and payment terms 2. guaranteed high quality work with emphasis on improvement 3. reduced administrative time relating to CRO selection for studies 4. dedicated staff for projects 5. reduced time to set up studies 6. reduced time to complete studies 7. innovation in clinical trial processes leading to reduced timing and improved quality

The Preferred Partnership concept is driven by three simple goals:

increased performance,
reduction in costs, and
innovation.

However, the substantial gains to be made from these arrangements will not be forthcoming unless a considerable effort is made by both parties to ensure that, at the evaluation, negotiation, and implementation stages, the commitment is clear and open.

At the CRO selection stage, the business needs of the client company must be defined and agreed to by all groups affected by the partnership. These business needs can vary considerably from seeking a partner for Phase I only, a partner for a single development project, or Phase II/III only for European studies to full service for the U.S.A., Europe and beyond. Agreement on these needs makes the selection and evaluation much easier because the target CROs will be different in each case. The level of outsourcing to be contracted must also be defined and agreed upon. CROs must be made aware of the amount of work to be contracted so that they can plan for staff and facilities required by the partnership.

Most important of all is that the partnership must be managed. There must be a commitment by the CRO to dedicate staff to work closely with the client and also a commitment of the client to dedicate staff to manage the partnership. As discussed in earlier sections, open, honest communications are essential to the smooth running of contracts, and this is even more important with a partnership. It is essential that combined planning meetings be held at specified intervals and that the progress of the partnership is monitored at the operational and strategic levels.

Several CROs have entered into preferred partnerships with clients, and some pharmaceutical companies and biotechnology companies have publicly announced the formation of such agreements. However, there is little published on the success of these arrangements within the pharmaceutical clinical research area, but, because other industries have documented benefits, it would be odd, indeed, if this were not so in the pharmaceutical industry. Over the next few years, we will learn whether the benefits expected have been generated.

Some observers have suggested that a preferred supplier relationship could make a CRO less willing or able to serve a sponsor which has not entered into such an agreement with the CRO. In fact, this is very unlikely in the current, highly competitive CRO marketplace. Each CRO must give each sponsor equivalent attention and a high standard of service to achieve and build success. CROs understand that small, early phase studies can grow into much larger, long-term projects and, therefore, demand focused attention. Moreover, no CRO, with or without a preferred provider agreement, wants to become too dependent on any one or even a few clients because major projects can easily fail or a sponsor's business strategies may suddenly change, leaving a highly dependent CRO vulnerable to an important, sudden loss of revenue.

V. RESPONSE BY CRO TO A REQUEST FOR A PROPOSAL

As described above, sponsors typically spend considerable time and resources in identifying and selecting CROs as candidates to carry out a project. Similarly CROs, now working in a highly competitive marketplace, must make every effort to be placed on a sponsor's list of candidates. This marketing process often includes advertising in trade and medical publications, direct mail campaigns to pharmaceutical and biotechnology companies, participation in exhibitions and technical programs at professional meetings and conventions, and periodic face-to-face meetings with sponsor representatives. Although these activities are important to assure name recognition by potential clients and to introduce key personnel, expertise and general service capabilities, nothing is as convincing as referral by clients satisfied by a CRO's performance on a project.

After preparing the list of CRO candidates being considered for a project, the sponsor issues a request for a proposal and budget quotation (RFP) to the CROs selected. Because project plans, resource requirements, and budget estimates vary greatly depending upon actual specifications, the sponsor must be explicit and detailed in defining expectations and requirements. Many pharmaceutical and biotechnology companies, which rely heavily on outsourcing for product research and development, have prepared highly detailed lists of activities for each component of a project, including the distribution of responsibility between the sponsor and CRO. When such a list is not available to a pharmaceutical company, experienced CROs provide an example to the sponsor to help define the scope of services required. The sponsor must recognize that the proposals and budgets from the responding CROs can be compared objectively only if each CRO is given the same specifications.

Assuming that an explicit RFP has been issued, the CROs' responses will depend on a variety of factors, including

Who prepares the proposal—In a smaller CRO, senior management and technical experts, who are typically involved in both operating and sales functions, contribute directly to the proposal and budget estimate. Larger CROs, with a more robust infrastructure and differentiated responsibilities, utilize dedicated proposal and budget development experts who obtain technical input from operating departments depending on the availability of documented prior company experience in the prospective project. Many experienced, sophisticated CROs utilize proven budget algorithms to prepare cost estimates for well-defined projects.

Operating experience and efficiencies—A CRO with substantial prior experience in a similar type project should be able to prepare a proposal and budget quotation reflecting the ability to recruit study investigators, conduct clinical monitoring, manage, analyze and interpret study data, and demonstrate efficiencies in the process.

Pricing decisions—The majority of mature CROs will prepare an initial budget estimate for the project from the best information available to them. In many instances, they may choose to submit this projection as the budget quotation, but a CRO might either decrease or increase this initial estimate prior to submitting it to the client. A decrease is most likely if the CRO expects that the competition for the work is intense or, in the worst case, if the CRO is desperate to win the project. (Desperation may indicate financial instability which will only deteriorate if the project is awarded at an insufficient budget.) On the other hand, a decision to increase a quotation, generally, recognizes that the project will encounter some specific challenges not previously realized or that the CRO cannot handle the project but can do so only by recruiting costly additional resources. Should a sponsor wish to award the project to a CRO which has provided either an apparently low or high quotation, the potential risks should be fully understood.

VI. PRELIMINARY BUDGET PROPOSALS

At times, sponsors request "ballpark" or "preliminary" budget quotations. Prior to responding, CROs must be certain they understand exactly what the sponsor is anticipating because the terms "ballpark" and "preliminary" may have either identical or vastly different definitions.

Ballpark estimates are generally considered to be very rough projections of cost for a project without final plans. Because ballpark quotations are typically subject to revision, it should be understood to be that they are "preliminary." Indeed, budget details for such projections are often limited to very broad categories of activity or service and are presented as a cost range (minimum to maximum).

Sponsors often request these ballpark estimates to assist them in preparing an initial budget for a project or an entire product development program. However, such an exercise is credible only if quantitative and qualitative parameters of work scope are defined in the proposal. Even when primary parameters are reasonably well described, it may be problematic to compare quotations among responding CROs because interpretation of the specifications, the depth of experience of the CROs, and the business strategy of each CRO vary in responding to the "ballpark" request. Sponsors must be prepared to accept substantial budget revisions as initial assumptions are modified in the final project plan.

In contrast to the preliminary "ballpark" estimate, sponsors may request a "preliminary" quotation, based on highly definitive criteria, to appoint a CRO at an early stage in the project. In such a situation, each CRO candidate is expected to prepare a definitive project implementation plan and budget quotation based on the specified criteria. Accordingly, the sponsor can compare the proposals and select a CRO before the final project plan has been defined. In fact, a sponsor may require the specific expertise and resources of the selected CRO to finalize the plan prior to implementation. In such a scenario, the CRO is expected to prepare a final budget quotation after the project plan and scope of work are fully defined.

CROs have also come to understand that sponsors may obtain "preliminary," yet definitive, quotations in deciding whether to utilize in-house or CRO resources for a project. Although CROs may not be delighted with this practice, they must recognize that a sponsor's internal resources are a competitor, as are other CROs, for most projects.

VII. PREPARING A FULLY COSTED PROPOSAL

Upon receiving a request for a proposal from a sponsor, each responding CRO should assure that they fully understand the specifications. If not, the sponsor should be contacted for clarification. Most sponsors are prepared to provide additional essential information if requested. Indeed, in some instances, the sponsor advises all CRO candidates of important clarifying information even though only one CRO has made the request. This helps to assure the sponsor that the proposals are directly comparable.

Although the proposal and budget quotation, in all likelihood, is not the only criterion used by the sponsor to select the CRO, they are pivotal. Accordingly, the proposal should be of high substantive and organizational quality, and the budget estimate must be objective and easily understood. At a minimum, the winning proposal must convincingly present the CRO's

  relevant therapeutic experience,
  staff and, where appropriate, consultant expertise,
  relevant project operational experience, for example, specific processes
      and systems for handling Phase I or large scale (> 50 centers, > 1000
      patients) studies,

specific plan for managing, designing, and implementing the project including a clear description of relevant capabilities, resources, information management systems and special technologies, such as remote data entry, interactive voice response systems, etc.,
quality assurance plan,
client communication and reporting plan, and
itemized budget estimate.

The proposal can be interpreted as an example of the quality of a CRO's services. Therefore, it is imperative that this document is submitted on time, addresses all sponsor specifications, is well organized, easily readable, and complete, yet succinct.

Proposals and budgets may be prepared via different means and individuals among CROs. However, in most instances, experts within functional groups or departments (for example, medical, regulatory, biostatistics, etc.) will be requested to provide specialized technical information for incorporation into the proposal. These professional experts should also be capable of projecting the types and quantities of human resources required for each task. These projections typically form the basis for detailed, objective budget preparation by expert budget or financial analysts.

The process of proposal and budget preparation may progressively become automated as experience grows within a CRO. When this occurs, each proposal should continue to receive appropriate professional input and review to assure accuracy, completeness, and sensitivity to the sponsor's requirements. To facilitate the retrieval and documentation of a CRO's therapeutic experience and staff expertise for multiple proposals, it is important for the CRO to develop user-friendly, relational databases of the company's study experience and staff expertise.

For many of the larger CROs, some form of automated project budget preparation has become essential to handle over a thousand quotations annually. These methodologies may also interface with human resource, project management, financial tracking, and sponsor reporting tools activated by project award and implementation.

Before a sponsor awards the work to any one of the responding CROs, generally, proposal presentation meetings are arranged by the sponsor with each of the competing CROs which appear most appropriate for the project based on the submitted proposals and, possibly, reference or other historical information. These sessions are critical in the selection process in terms of the substance of the discussions and the participants. Ideally, the client should visit the "short-listed" CROs to meet as many of the key, potential project team members as possible and evaluate facilities, SOPs and applicable technologies and systems. Although CRO visits at sponsor facilities are more convenient and cost-efficient for the sponsor in the short run, they are likely to be less informative to the sponsor and, perhaps, most costly in the long term if the wrong CRO is selected because of insufficient insight into the CRO's infrastructure, expertise, systems, and operating philosophies.

Ultimately, the winning CRO will have convinced the sponsor to make the selection, in large part, based on the proposal and quotation submitted, the caliber of the project team, the quality and content of the face-to-face meeting(s), demonstrated project-specific experience and systems, past project performance, financial stability of the company, and reference checks.

In summary, the winning proposal and associated discussions will have

identified the key personnel for the project,
defined the details of the activities to be carried out,
agreed on task distribution between sponsor and CRO,
established and agreed explicit timelines,
agreed on a definitive budget structure to avoid unexpected extra costs,
considered time and cost efficiencies while assuring quality,
established performance targets,
established communication channels and frequencies, and
assured that all sponsor specifications have been addressed.

VIII. ACTIONS FOLLOWING PROPOSAL AWARD

A. Actions Within the CRO

CRO selection may require one to three months, possibly delaying the initiation of a project. To avoid any further delay, the sponsor and selected CRO must negotiate a contract promptly or, at a minimum, agree to proceed under a letter of intent.

Sponsors, who outsource considerable amounts of work, often have prototype contracts available which define standard terms and conditions for CRO services. Alternatively, the CRO may propose an initial draft to begin the negotiation. In either case, assuming that the parties agree with the proposed contract terms and the proposal can readily be incorporated into the contract via reference, the project can get underway immediately.

In the event that contract development extends beyond the project start date, a letter of intent often suffices to initiate the work. Such a letter typically authorizes the CRO to conduct a specific portion of the planned project over a defined period of time for an agreed cost. The sponsor and CRO should make every effort to reach a contract during the period covered by the letter of intent to avoid further delays and assure that neither party is inappropriately exposed to business risks and liabilities. The entire process of CRO selection and contract negotiation can be streamlined greatly through preferred provider or master service agreements (see below).

Although agreement on the scope of work, the associated timelines, and the budget is usually straightforward, arriving at an appropriate payment schedule may be more difficult. The costs commonly defined as indirect or pass-through, such as investigator and laboratory payments and travel and lodging costs for CRO monitoring personnel, are often treated separately from direct or CRO personnel costs. The indirect costs are often paid by the sponsor through an initial installment to cover start-up expenses followed by periodic payments for invoices submitted by the CRO. Although sponsors also commonly agree to make an up-front payment for start-up activities of the CRO's project team, agreement on a payment schedule thereafter can be much more challenging.

Sponsors recognize that CROs and investigators alike cannot be expected to fund the pharmaceutical company's research and, therefore, are aware that these service providers must be paid appropriately. At the same time, sponsors wish to hold CROs and investigators accountable and, accordingly, would like to pay for performance. Overall, this is a fully acceptable approach, assuming that the performance milestones on which the sponsor wishes to make payments are controlled by the service provider. Payment schedules, which are primarily based on the number of patients enrolled in a difficult clinical trial, may be considered unreasonable or even punitive by a CRO, if, for example,

the CRO is not responsible for selecting the clinical investigators,
the patient selection criteria in the sponsor's study protocol are too
   limiting to allow timely patient recruitment, or
the timeline for patient enrollment is unrealistically short.

On the other hand, payment schedules based solely on fixed dates may be considered unacceptable to sponsors unless the contract incorporates other performance measures to assure that the CRO is using best efforts to accomplish the task. Alternatively, payment schedules that require some type of risk sharing between the sponsor and CRO may be appropriate. This approach might require that the sponsor pays the CRO on a fixed-date-certain basis, but the CRO has to forfeit profit if work performance is inadequate; this lost profit could be recovered later if the CRO brings the project back on schedule. Ultimately, the payment schedule and contract as a whole should target a win-win outcome for both sponsor and CRO.

Upon formal authorization to begin work, the CRO must establish the project team. Frequently, core members of the team will already have been identified and introduced to the sponsor during the final selection process and the full complement of staff will become involved in accordance with the proposal as their support is required.

An initial or project launch meeting which requires the active participation of key team members from both the sponsor and CRO is essential for project success. This session should result in a practical understanding of the following:

> Features of an initial project launch meeting:
> the development status of the project under study,
> project scope and detailed plans for implementation,
> protocol and other study documents,
> assignments of responsibility and authority,
> regulatory requirements,
> time lines,
> contract terms (if agreed),
> lines and methods of communication,
> performance measures,
> team member training plans,
> operating procedures for key activities, such as serious adverse event
>   reporting, clinical monitoring and data management guidelines, and
>   criteria for releasing drug supply,
> reporting requirements,
> quality assurance plans, etc.

In essence, the entire team must leave the meeting with a common recognition of objectives and how they will be achieved.

In concert with the launch meeting or at another early point during project initiation, protocol-specific training should be provided to clinical monitors, data managers, and other critical members of the team. Medically qualified representatives from both the sponsor and CRO are often required to take a central role in this training. The clinical monitors, who will be interacting with study investigators, must have a good understanding of the disease or condition being treated, the product being evaluated, the types of data being collected, and any data review conventions or criteria which the data managers and statisticians will be using. Because data managers generally must review the completed case record forms, resolve queries through the support of the clinical monitors, and build study databases for statistical analysis, it may be ideal to train monitors and data managers simultaneously.

B. Actions Within the Sponsor

One of the major problems encountered frequently following the decision to award a contract to a particular CRO is the negotiation of the contract and the question of a letter of intent. It should be remembered that the contract between the sponsor and CRO consists of several distinct parts and the responsibility for compiling the parts rests with different people. The typical principal Terms and Conditions of a contract and those responsible for their completion are listed below:

parties and definitions	legal
definition and performance of services	legal/clinical
price and payment	legal/clinical/finance
confidentiality	legal
ownership	legal
data, publication, and intellectual property	legal/clinical
status of the parties	legal
compensation and indemnity	legal
terms and termination	legal/clinical

Under each of the major headings are several subheadings which need expert legal input. For example, under the heading of confidentiality are clauses on the definition of confidentiality, nondisclosure, return of confidential materials, terms of the obligation, and disclosure and ownership of intellectual property. Because of the importance of the legal contract, most pharmaceutical companies ensure that their clinical research staff has available standard "boiler plate" sections covering the legally drafted sections of the contract. However, for those companies who do not have this facility, a contract should be drafted for them by companies which specialize in pharmaceutical contracting. It is also useful to append the detailed Price and Payment Schedule and Protocol and Procedures Manual to the Contract. There will be occasions when the CRO suggests that the sponsor use their contract. For those pharmaceutical companies which do not have a standard contract for these purposes, this can be an advantage and will save time. However, the contract must be reviewed by the company Legal Department or by an independent expert. Therein lies a problem. Legal consideration can take time and points raised may appear trivial, on occasion, but they must be resolved before the contract can be signed. Anyone who has contracted for a study with the prestigious universities and medical schools on the U.S. East Coast will understand the dialogue which can ensue following a minor disagreement about a contract. The signature on the contract must be appropriately chosen, as it will be considered legally binding by the CRO. Thus, it must be determined who within the sponsor has the authority to commit the company to a contract and at what level of funding. Although the effort is directed to drafting and agreeing on the contract, the CRO will be keen to start the preliminary activities needed if they are to meet the sponsor's deadlines. The sponsor will also want to see some progress. At this juncture, the possibility of issuing a letter of intent will be raised. It has to be understood that a letter of intent or even a "comfort letter" can be legally binding and should be issued with great care. However, when used prudently and with clear points stating what can be done under the letter of intent, it can be most useful. It should also be remembered that the authorization issue raised earlier applies to these letters in addition to the contracts.

A vital ingredient to ensuring the success for a contract is good, open, and honest communication between the CRO and the sponsor. During the CRO selection phase, a team within the sponsor will have been active in evaluating the bidding companies. Once the contract has been awarded or during the drafting, it is vital that those team members do not think that their job is done. A team must be maintained and must meet with their counterparts within the CRO at a frequency agreeable to both parties. It must be made clear to these staff that they have a continuing role to play and must devote time to the monitoring and management of the contract. All team members from the sponsor and CRO must be given defined roles and must clearly understand their responsibilities, accountabilities, and time schedules. It is good practice to nominate a point person within each company to act as a first contact when any issues are to be raised. A system of progress review must be agreed on and a reporting schedule confirmed. There are many opinions expressed as to the internal resource required of a sponsor to monitor and manage successfully a contracted study. This will depend on the scale and complexity of the study but has been put by some authorities as high as one-third of the staff resource employed on the contract by the CRO. This may be extreme, but it illustrates the importance of sponsor involvement even when studies are contracted out. There will be some areas where the sponsor will wish to issue and agree on written guidelines for the CRO to follow. Most notably, these will relate to reporting of serious adverse events; the flow of information, responsibility for action, and reporting being clearly documented and agreed upon. Other areas where it is important to have written agreements are in the criteria for release of drug supply, and data management guidelines. Once these are agreed to, then, they should become part of the written contract as an appendix along with the protocol.

There is debate about the most appropriate level of sponsor management of contracts. For a short Phase I study enrolling a small number of healthy subjects, which is not a first administration-to-human study, it would probably be unreasonable to micro manage the study. However, for a difficult multinational Phase III study, it is not uncommon for the sponsor and CRO to be in daily contact. This involvement, if spelled out at the onset of the contract discussions, should not be seen as a burden by the CRO but welcomed as a measure of the involvement and commitment of the sponsor to the study.

It is often overlooked that the progress of the contracted study should be communicated within the sponsor. Senior management has a right to be kept up to date with progress or problems. Good, open, honest communication between sponsor and CRO during all stages of a contract, before and after the award, will ensure that no "nasty" surprises occur.

IX. WHAT TO DO IF IT ALL GOES WRONG

A. The Pharmaceutical Company Perspective

Even with all the careful planning and optimism at the start of a contract, there will be occasions when things will go wrong. Patient enrollment may be affected by seasonal variability, or staff changes within CRO, the sponsor, or the investigator site can adversely effect the smooth running of the contract; drop out rates are higher than anticipated or a flood results in the loss of patient records at a major site. Clearly some problems cannot be anticipated, and not all problems occur because of a fault within the CRO or sponsor. However, it is prudent at the onset of a project to identify and discuss possible problem areas which are generic to clinical research and development. It is also good practice to have contingency plans for the more obvious problems which might occur. This will save considerable time and effort and, hopefully, resolve issues without missing vital agreed milestones. Any hint of a problem must be communicated immediately by the CRO to the sponsor and vice versa. It is important that, along with reporting the possibility of a problem, the CRO and sponsor should propose solutions, showing that the CRO is committed to the same goals as the sponsor. If the problem was foreseen, then, a solution may be found quickly, but, if the problem was not anticipated, an early proposal for resolving it will benefit both parties.

If the CRO and sponsor have worked openly and honestly during the development of the contract, then, as long as problems have arisen through circumstances, not from faulty performance by the CRO or sponsor, then, it should be possible to resolve them quickly and amicably.

Unfortunately, however, there will still be cases where it is deemed that the problem has arisen because of poor performance by the CRO. In these cases, it is best to work together to resolve the problem. Most agreements will provide a period during which, having received written notice of a deficiency, the CRO will have time to correct the fault. If the fault cannot be rectified to the sponsor's satisfaction, then there may be no alternative but to terminate the contract and transfer the study to the sponsor or to another CRO. This is so time consuming and wasteful that all efforts should be made before this drastic step.

Working together before the contract is awarded, being open and honest during negotiation, being prepared to spend the time to manage the contract, and having contingency plans for possible problems should protect both the sponsor and CRO from the results of contract termination.

B. Project Management Within the CRO

Objective, continuous review and proactive communication are always the key to dealing with problems in the course of conducting a project. Clinical research involves people and processes which, by definition, are not always predictable. Whether a project is conducted by the pharmaceutical company alone or through a CRO, problems or unexpected challenges will likely arise. This must be acknowledged by the two parties from the outset. Ideally, the entire team, sponsor and CRO included, must be committed to the same goals of success.

The project team should be aware of and, in some cases, document the problems anticipated during the project. This exercise includes identifying contingency plans. Whether or not problems have been anticipated, solutions, should be proposed by the CRO when problems occur, rather than simply reporting the event or situation. Moreover, problematic issues should be addressed as soon as possible to minimize negative outcomes and maintain the confidence of the entire team.

Pharmaceutical product development, generally, depends on multidisciplinary project teams. Depending on the needs of the pharmaceutical

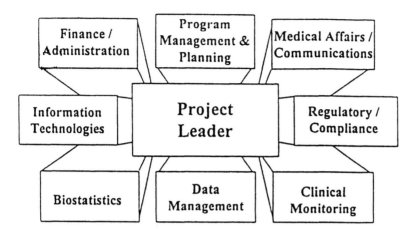

FIG. 1   Project team.

sponsor, a CRO may be requested to provide support in a single discipline, such as clinical monitoring or statistical analysis, or may be required to contribute a full range of disciplines as depicted in Fig. 1.

To respond adequately and flexibly in addressing the highly variable needs of multiple sponsors in terms of project size, scope, and therapeutic discipline, most major CROs employ a matrix management system. This approach requires that team members are drawn from technical departments to serve the specific needs of a project under the leadership of a project manager.

In this management structure, the team members report to the project manager on a dotted line basis while maintaining direct reporting responsibility to their respective technical departments. Ideally, this assures consistent, high-quality technical support from each discipline across multiple projects throughout the CRO, while demanding expert leadership and management from each project manager. The project manager is typically a member of a project management department which provides training, management guidance, tools and ancillary resources to each manager.

Historically, pharmaceutical companies often expected medical doctors or other scientists to lead and manage projects. However, over time, the management component of that responsibility has gradually shifted to individuals of various backgrounds who have been specifically trained to lead and manage people and operational processes. In this way, physicians and scientists, who might not have a strong interest in or aptitude for managerial activities, can maximize their professional contribution to each project while leaving management to expert managers. This is fully consistent with the CRO's approach.

Because the CRO's project manager is generally responsible for primary communication with the sponsor's project leader, the project manager has a major influence on the success of the relationship between sponsor and CRO. Consequently, the manager assigned to a project is becoming an increasingly important determinant in the selection of a CRO by a sponsor.

Beginning with a launch meeting, as described above, the CRO's project manager must assure that all activities associated with the project have been identified and scheduled and that appropriate staff has been assigned to each task. Integral to the implementation process is the verification that the plan presented to the sponsor in the initial proposal is fully consistent with the sponsor's actual requirements. Substantive variations which have budget impact should be fully documented, budgeted, and approved by the sponsor to avoid misunderstandings during the project. Notably, the entire project team (sponsor and CRO) must understand and adopt the work plan to assure project success.

The CRO project manager must track project progress relative to the plan and report to the sponsor on a periodic basis, perhaps, as frequently as weekly and at least monthly. This evaluation of progress should be accompanied monthly by a financial review to assure that actual costs are consistent with the approved budget and that operational efficiencies are maintained.

The CRO project manager must communicate with the sponsor on all primary project initiatives and status and must also assure appropriate communication throughout the project team to coordinate the overall function of the team.

It is often essential that functional departments within the CRO, such as clinical monitoring, medical, or regulatory, communicate directly with their sponsor counterparts. In such an event, the project managers (CRO and sponsor) should be advised of any key decisions to assure that the project plan and/or budget will not be affected. If a change in work scope and budget are required, this should be documented formally and in a timely manner by the project manager and submitted to the sponsor for approval. A graphic representation of this typical communication model is shown in Fig. 2.

As discussed above, problems are likely to arise during the course of a project. Undoubtedly, the project manager will be required to take a

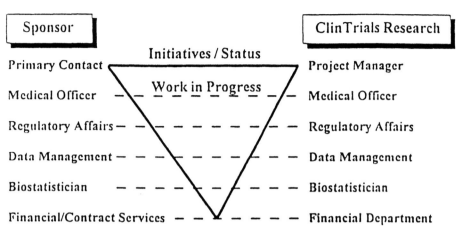

FIG. 2 Communication model.

proactive role in addressing these situations with the sponsor and assuring that the project team takes appropriate action. The CRO, which is concerned about continuous improvement of service to all clients, will document each substantive issue and its resolution, thereby, creating a database for future reference by project teams.

The lessons learned in each project should be reviewed with the sponsor and the CRO's project team periodically during an extended study and at the time of completion. This exercise will support process improvement in each organization and should help build a long-term relationship between the parties.

As in many settings of contemporary human interaction, the negative experiences of a sponsor/CRO collaboration are often given most attention, and inordinate amounts of time and effort may be directed to finding fault. Far greater benefit will accrue to both sponsors and CROs by examining what worked and how to avoid negative experiences in the future. Numerous professional meetings and publications have addressed relationships between sponsor and CRO that have or have not been successful [3,4]. Past and future open forums are sure to be helpful guides to sponsors and CROs embarking on new collaborations.

REFERENCES

1. AJ Siemens, J.E. Higgins, The Role of Clinical Research Organizations in Drug Development, The Drug Development Process. Marcel Dekker, New York, 1996, p. 337–352.
2. G Hughes, Drug Information Association Meeting, Orlando, Florida 1995.
3. FR Mangan, The Practicalities of Successfully Evaluating CROs for Preferred Provider Contracts to Enable You to Make the Best Choice of Partner for Your Organization, IIR Meeting, December 1995, London.
4. FR Mangan, Objectively Evaluating CROs for Partnerships and New Approaches to Obtain Competitive Bids, IIR Meeting, December 1994, London.

8

Project Managing: The Development of Drug Delivery Devices

Alec MacAndrew

Cambridge Technology Centre
Melbourn, Hertsfordshire, England

I. WHY DEVICES FOR DRUG DELIVERY?

In an ideal world, there would be no need for drug delivery devices. In this Utopia, all drugs would be perfectly efficacious, free of side effects, and delivered orally. In reality, many drugs cannot be delivered orally, are more efficacious, or have less severe side effects if they are delivered by an alternative route.

Alternative routes of administration are preferred because of the particular characteristics of the molecule or the indication. For example, first-pass metabolism, low bioavailability in the gastrointestinal tract, the need for topical action, and systemic side effects are all phenomena which dictate alternative routes of administration. Consequently, many drugs must be delivered or are better delivered, for example, by injection, inhalation, implantation, or transdermally. The devices with access to these routes, such as injectors, IV systems, inhalers, IUDs, iontophoretic patches and so on, are being developed in numbers greater than ever before.

II. THE CHANGING DEVICE BUSINESS

The time has passed when pharmaceutical companies could regard these devices as the sole province of device suppliers: companies which develop, manufacture, and market standard products. Of course, the need for off-the-shelf devices remains, and the device supply industry is growing and becoming more sophisticated. Pharmaceutical companies, however, must regard customized devices optimized for their individual needs as a priority. There are several reasons for this:

- Increasingly, new chemical entities which require nonoral administration are being developed in conjunction with the delivery device, so that the complete development links the drug and the device development programs, and the drug and device combination can be regarded as the complete product.
- Devices often provide positive differentiating factors which promote a competitive advantage for the pharmaceutical company. Examples abound, but some of the more well known include Astra's Turbuhaler®, the insulin injector pens of Novo and other diabetes care companies, Glaxo-Wellcome's inhalers and its antimigraine injection device, and smoking cessation patches and inhalers.
- Regulatory requirements and the needs of patients cause substantial customization, even of catalogue devices, and the modifications to satisfy the pharmaceutical company's needs for particular dose size

and accuracy or special features result in a substantial product development program linked to the drug development program.

The consequence of the closer meshing between the development of drug substance and the device to deliver it is that the same pressures on time to market and regulatory compliance apply equally to drug and device. In spite of all this, device development is still frequently perceived within the pharmaceutical industry as easier than drug development and as somewhat peripheral to the core business.

It is natural for the head of pharmaceutical development to underestimate the difficulty (if not the importance) of developing an excellent drug delivery device. It is extremely hard to imagine, without painful experience, what pitfalls lie in disciplines other than one's own, and no head of pharmaceutical development is likely to be a mechanical engineer, a physicist, or a designer.

Underestimating the difficulty or size of the device development project can lead to several undesirable consequences:

*   selection of an inappropriate organization to conduct the development, either under-qualified or under-resourced
*   inadequate or nonexistent management of the project
*   poor management of risk
*   poor integration of the many functions required to launch a successful device
*   separation of the drug development from the device development program.

The result of falling into these traps is often disaster with, at best, substantial delays to the launch of the product and, at worst, cancellation of the development. If we have stressed the risks associated with treating device development too lightly, it is because experience shows that it is the underlying cause for many severe development problems. So, what can be done in project management to maximize the chance of success?

III. SELECTING A DEVELOPMENT RESOURCE

Selecting the right team to undertake development of the device is the critical first step in the process. Recognizing the full range of skills needed often comes as a shock. Skills needed in many projects include mechanical engineering and design; electronics; software; ergonomics and industrial design; analytical chemistry; materials science; production engineering; tool development; drug formulation and development pharmacy; pharmacology; clinical research; regulatory affairs; packaging; production line design; assembly and filling equipment design; production validation; market research and marketing. This long (but not exhaustive) list can result in two challenges. First, there is often difficulty in assembling all the skills at the right time. Second, the project manager faces a real challenge in pulling all of these disparate strands together.

It is unusual that any single organization has every skill in-house. The challenge lies not just in creating an internal structure with representatives of all the disciplines, but in maintaining those skills at the leading edge of practice and in providing a career structure for people with minority skills. The answer is to form a collaborative team from a number of different organizations, each of which is expert and competent in one or several of the key disciplines. In other words, outsourcing of some elements is usually necessary.

Choosing the members of the team is the first important step in the development process and, critically important, because the success of the project depends on it. Each organization contributing to the collaboration should possess one or a number of core skills and have sufficient knowledge of the others' contributions to interact effectively. It is no good engaging the very best design house if it has no people with experience or knowledge of the vagaries and subtleties of the drug/device interaction.

If going it alone is often inadvisable, having too many different organizations contributing to the development can also be a mistake. The challenge of communicating and coordinating across the project team requires a limited number of primary collaborators. Experience shows that it is easy to lose control with more than three. Of course, there is no reason why any of the primary contributors should not engage and manage specialist subcontract services.

There are three broad categories of skill required to develop a device:

- analytical chemistry, drug formulation, clinical research, regulatory affairs and marketing which are usually best undertaken by a pharmaceutical company (although outsourcing of some of these elements is possible and increasingly likely)
- assembly and filling line development; molding and tool making are usually undertaken by a specialist GMP manufacturing company. Some elements (particularly filling and final assembly) frequently remain the responsibility of the pharmaceutical partner
- the design, consisting of industrial design and ergonomics, mechanical engineering and design, electronics, software, and so forth.

TABLE 1

Selection of a Design Resource: Pharmaceutical Company

Development resource	Advantages	Disadvantages
Pharmaceutical company	• Use of in-house resources • Confidentiality • Clear ownership of intellectual property • Control	• Lack of skills/resources • Time • Inexperience in device development • Noncore business

TABLE 2

Selection of a Design Resource: Manufacturing Partner

Development resource	Advantages	Disadvantages

Manufacturing partner	• Potentially lower development costs
	• Intimate knowledge of molding
	• Seamless integration between development and manufacturing
		• Locked in
		• Potential for intellectual property confusion
		• Absence of core product development skills
		• Vested interests
		  —molding weight cost
		  —design authority
		• Confidentiality

TABLE 3

Selection of a Design Resource: Specialist Product Development Organization

Development resource	Advantages	Disadvantages
Specialist product development organization	• Clear ownership of intellectual property • Special expertise in device development • Application of key skills • Minimum manufacturing cost • High-quality design • Confidentiality	• Up-front development costs • More parties involved

This last function can be the responsibility of the pharmaceutical company, the manufacturing partner, or a specialist product development organization. Each approach has its own advantages and disadvantages, and the choice depends on individual circumstances. Tables 1, 2, and 3 show some of the advantages and disadvantages of each approach.

IV. MANAGEMENT OF DIVERSE PROJECT RESOURCES

The first step has been taken, and a competent team is in place. What does the project manager have to do to manage the resource?

The very diversity of skills needed to carry out a device development causes the first headache for the project manager, to coordinate this wide range of input, to ensure that the entire team is working to the same schedules, that all to be done is being done, and that activities are not being duplicated.

Very importantly, the project manager must understand enough about each of the many disciplines to coordinate them and to act as a facilitator for their often conflicting requirements. This does not mean that the project manager must be a competent practitioner in all (or indeed in any) of them, but he must speak many technical languages and act as a conduit and interpreter of information between different disciplines. Avoiding the "Tower of Babel" effect is a prime responsibility.

For example, if there is a need to facilitate a debate between the formulation chemist, the materials scientist and the toolmaker on alternative solutions to, say, a dose uniformity problem, the project manager must understand the meaning of such concepts as excipients and micronization, the triboelectric series and plastic deformation, and hot runners and ejector pins. Real problems arise on projects at the interfaces, particularly where one discipline underestimates or ignores the need for another. The project manager must ensure that the needs and constraints of each party are understood by the others to the extent needed to make the best decision for the project.

This facility to understand and debate with all disciplines is the most important skill the device development project manager can have and one of the most difficult to acquire. It comes only through experience and an insatiable desire to learn applied across all the disciplines. It is destroyed by the fatal assumption that any one or two skills are much more important to the development than others.

V. THE MAKEUP OF THE PROJECT TEAM

Project teams are not and should not be static institutions, established on day one and set in stone for the duration of the project.

Many developments begin with an invention or some other piece of creative thinking. The management of the transition from invention to full product development must take account of the fact that inventors of device concepts are often not good at developing detailed and robust engineering solutions. This issue can arise both with in-house and with licensed-in concepts and, if not managed well, can be troublesome or fatal later.

The makeup of the team should change according to the development stage. Inventors, naturally, feel strong ownership for their creation and sometimes fail to recognize their deficiencies. In this case, the goal of the project manager must be to retain the creativity, commitment, and experience of the inventor while moving the design responsibility to a results-focused professional development team. One good approach is to retain the inventor as advisor or guru, but not in such a rôle where he can single handedly override the design authority that the project manager has vested in the development team. This needs a degree of tact usually to be found only in career diplomats.

Similarly with the rest of the development, the project manager must engage and disengage different skills at the appropriate time during the development. In many cases, getting the right people when they are most needed requires careful planning and persistence.

For many skills, the appropriate time to be engaged is earlier than has conventionally been the case. Input from component manufacturers and from those responsible for assembly, filling, testing, packaging, and marketing the product should not be left to the end. The best devices are easy to mold, easy to assemble, easy to fill, work well with the drug, and meet the market needs, and this cannot be achieved by ignoring these aspects to the last minute. The project management challenge is to engage downstream skills early enough and to ensure that they are seen as full team members and that their input is heeded. It is more difficult to coordinate bigger teams with sometimes conflicting demands, so the temptation is strong to keep the team small and easily managed. Nevertheless, experience across industry shows that overall quality and timescales are enhanced by getting parallel input early, compared with the conventional serial approach.

VI. PHASING THE PROJECT

Parallel working does not mean that everyone does everything at once and that the project lacks structure.

Inexperienced device development managers often see the development as a single monolithic task. This, and thinking that the project is further advanced than it is, are major stumbling blocks. Time and time again, we come across attempts to initiate the manufacturing of designs which are no more refined than proof-of-principle models.

As the development progresses, the emphasis and the immediate objectives change. The planning and management of the project are enhanced immeasurably by dividing the development into phases and being clear about the objectives and the levels of hardware sophistication in each phase.

Figure 1 shows a project structure which, experience has shown, is suitable for developing drug delivery devices. All device developments, whether they are clean sheet projects taking five years from concept to launch or fast track developments of simple devices taking less than a year, go through these or very similar stages. Sometimes it is possible or desirable to take a short cut or eliminate a stage, but, then, it is dangerous to pretend that no short cut has been taken and it is as well to acknowledge that the technical risk is increased.

Massive short cutting, generally, is a false economy. So is the monolithic concept of design, where there are no planned design iterations. In this case, the initial project schedule often seems seductively short. The reality is that this approach results in unplanned and seemingly endless design modifications, a configuration out of control, unmanageable risk, and often, failure.

There are other models that can be used to structure the project. One does not have to use the model of Figure 1, but some structure should be used.

VII. MEETING CUSTOMERS' NEEDS

It is necessary, but not sufficient, that devices be safe and efficacious. They must be well designed, easy to use and, in the case of devices for patient self-administration, they should promote patient compliance. The cleverest and most advanced delivery concept can be let down by poor attention to the real clinical needs of health professionals and patients.

The project manager has the responsibility to ensure that industrial design is not an after thought. It is no good predicting what responses patients will have to different designs of device. Good quality research must be done to determine patients' and health professionals' views and to observe objectively how they cope with operating the proposed design of a device. The project manager has to curb the natural desire of the team to forge ahead without this information, and he must ensure that the lessons learned from patient and doctor acceptance trials are applied to the design.

Stage	Concept/Invention /Patent	Laboratory Demonstrator	Engineering Model	Prototype	Production Start-up	Production Ramp-up
What		Works like	Works identically Looks like	Works identically Looks identical Made like	Works identically Looks identical Made identically	Works identically Looks identical Made identically Assembled identically
Purpose		Demonstration of base function	**Demonstrates** - performance - key areas of risk **Defines** - budget costs - investment required - ergonomics - size/weight - modularity - appearance - basic design **Enables** - formulation development	**Demonstrates** - ergonomics - appearance - functionality - size/weight - reliability **Defines** - materials - manufacturing route - assembly & test - detailed design - unit cost - design for assembly **Enables** - clinical trials	**Demonstrates** -production tools -test facilities -assembly tooling -supplier capability -quality -process validation **Enables** - clinical trials - product launch	**Demonstrates** - complete assembly process - high volume - quality/yield/cost targets **Enables** - best cost production
Hardware	Rigs?	Functional - unlike a device	Fabricated & some soft tool parts	Prototype tools 1 million components if required	Production tools - limited quantities	Tools: Production

The process of determining customers' needs begins with good market research. All too often, "good" is interpreted to mean "extensive." The market for drug delivery cannot be researched in the same way as the market for washing powder. Better to concentrate on fewer influential respondents, particularly when seeking the views of health care professionals, and to ensure that the interviews thoroughly explore their views. The project manager has the difficult task of leading the Marketing Department and the technical experts on the team in translating the findings of market research into the first draft of the Product Requirement Specification.

Tools, such as Customer Preference Modeling, which allow more objective trade-offs between features and cost and between different features, should be used at this stage.

Research later in the project, in the form of acceptance trials with professionals and with patients, should always use tangible stimulus material. This should take the form of more or less realistic models of different concepts for meeting the Requirements Specification, which respondents can comment on and which can be used to explore how well users cope with operating the device. For a device for self-administration, patients should receive about the same level of training and explanation as they would in a real clinical setting, and their subsequent attempts to use the device models can be recorded on video for later analysis.

The project manager should be the conscience of the team. He has to ensure that the optimal concept is chosen, based on the findings of the trial, rather than on the prejudices of the team, which do not always coincide. The project manager also has to encourage the team to solve real issues which arise from the research and to avoid the temptation of sweeping these problems under the carpet. For example, a majority of patient respondents might criticize the procedure for reloading the device, and this might well be supported by the practical evidence based on their attempts to do so with the models during the interview. To ignore these findings and to rationalize the issue away by asserting that patients will learn in time to cope would be a big mistake and would result in a substantially poorer device than if the difficult task of solving the ergonomic difficulty was faced.

VIII. THE PRODUCT REQUIREMENT SPECIFICATION

Good devices have been launched without ever having a formal Product Requirement Specification but that is just good luck.

Professionally managed device development should have a Requirement Specification in place before the start of the Engineering Model phase.

This specification should be based on prior experience and good market research, because this is the only way to ensure that everyone on the team has the same concept of what the device must be, that the concept supports the market requirements, and that the temptation of creeping elegance is avoided. The Requirements Specification is a living document and can be changed. However, the change should be made consciously and with full understanding of the implications for project duration and risk. A certain degree of inertia is a good thing, so that change requires some effort. The inertia should increase as the assignment progresses, so that changes to the Requirement Specification become almost impossible as the preparation of clinical trial material approaches. All affected by changes should agree to them and sign them off.

The project manager is the keeper of the Requirement Specification. This means that the project manager has to negotiate and interpret conflicting needs and document their resolution in the Specification. The project manager must also ensure that the design meets the Specification and is shown to do so by arranging different types of testing. If the device fails to meet the Requirement Specification, the project manager must make the team face this and resolve it explicitly by improving the performance of the device or by accepting the deficiency formally by changing the Specification.

IX. TESTING

There are three broad categories of device testing; mechanical and life testing, analytical testing, and clinical testing.

Because it is outside normal pharmaceutical practice, mechanical testing is often ignored. The project manager should ensure that the device is tested properly for robustness and that the tests represent the most severe environments that the device will encounter in the glove compartments of motor cars, in handbags and pockets, and across the globe from Scandinavia in winter to a tropical paradise.

The need for analytical testing to support the in vitro investigation of the device's functionality is well understood. The critical tasks for the project manager are to ensure an adequate test plan, provide sufficient resources, and establish protocols which are followed. Analytical testing is often on the critical path, particularly when technical problem solving is underway. A big mistake, frequently made, is to treat the analytical test resource as an external service rather than as an integral part of the development team. In the midst of a major technical problem, the test plan can change on a daily basis ("Let's carry out test A on five devices and, if we find result X, then, we carry out test B on five more devices, whereas, if we get result Y, then, we modify five devices and repeat test A..." etc.) and the team will not get the necessary commitment from a service function.

Clinical testing is usually the greatest and the least of the project manager's headaches. It is the greatest in the sense that getting there on time with a good device doing what it is meant to do is, perhaps, the major challenge for the project manager and the objective at which much of his effort is aimed. It is least in the sense that once there with a good device, an efficacious molecule, and a well designed trial, the rest should fall into place.

X. TOOLS

A wide range of tools is available for managing all types of projects. Many general tools are relevant to drug device development and ought to be used by the project manager. We shall concentrate on commenting on some key tools for device development.

A. The Project Plan

The project plan is the primary tool of project control and an important means of communication with the team. The huge range of skills and functions needed to develop a successful device make planning even more important than in other projects. The availability of planning tools for personal computers, such as MS Project and MacProject, has made the professional planner redundant in many situations. In one respect, direct control of the plan by the team members is a good thing because it promotes ownership, commitment, and the ability to change the plan quickly and easily as circumstances demand. On the other hand, the use of this tool is a skill that must be acquired, not just in respect to the technical aspects of using the tool but also in the ability to draw together diverse and interdependent activities in a logical and consistent manner (in other words, to think like a planner). Bad planning can be worse than no planning at all.

There should be a top level plan which shows, in outline, all the activities for the complete development. There should be more detailed plans for each project phase, and within those, yet more detailed plans for individual functions. The detailed plans should reflect the requirements of the higher level plan but should feed back into it so that the questions "What do we have to do?" and "What have we got time to do?" receive the right balance of emphasis depending on the relative priorities of functionality and timescales. The plans together should form a self consistent set.

A good device project manager should be conversant with the use of network (PERT-type) and bar (Gantt-type) schedules. The PERT-type is invaluable for understanding the complex interrelationships between the many functions and disciplines involved in developing the device. The Gantt-type is clearer for timescale, overlap and slack within the project and represents the better format for management reporting.

Where several organizations are involved in a development, it is essential that they all work to the same schedule. This can be achieved only if they all have access to the same software planning tool and regularly share their thinking on scheduling. The plans of each contributing party, particularly where they interact, should be consistent. All too often, we see quite well-structured plans for individual functions which demand the impossible or fail to deliver the essential information to the rest of the team. This should be avoided by proper integration in the top-level plan.

A common pitfall is to consider the planning job done once the schedules are written. Plans are the most effective way to ensure timely delivery, by tracking at least weekly, often daily, and sometimes hourly. If the project manager looks after the hours and days, the years will take care of themselves.

B. Failure Modes and Effects Analysis

Failure Modes and Effects Analysis (FMEA) is a technique which originated in the aerospace and nuclear industries where successful performance first time is important. The method is to use prior experience, to brainstorm, or otherwise to predict in any way possible how the device and its interaction with the drug, its assembly, and filling can go wrong. The likelihood and effect of such a failure, then, is predicted. Failure modes, particularly where they are deemed to be likely and where the effect is severe, are then avoided by redesign or by some other means. By following this process, a more robust device results. A certain level of FMEA, properly documented, is required within Europe to acquire the CE mark.

C. The Design Review

Good practice calls for regular, independent design reviews during the project. All sorts of embarrassing problems to do with fit and function can be avoided by recognizing them early enough. Employing a fresh pair (or several fresh pairs) of eyes to look critically at the project helps to flush out problems that the team cannot or will not see. The scope of independent reviews can be to cover the entire project in all its aspects including both process (planning, management, coordination, etc.) and content (design, engineering, manufacture, drug/device interaction, and so on). The reviews can help to identify problems and to suggest solutions. The ideal reviewer is familiar with the basic project objectives, unconnected with the detailed content or process of the project (thus, independent and fresh), and expert and experienced in carrying out similar projects (and so, best qualified to spot potential or real problems and to offer good advice).

D. Technical Tools

The team can use a vast array of tools that carry out each individual function effectively. These include Design for Manufacturing; Design for Assembly; Value Engineering; Finite Elements Analysis; Mold Flow Analysis; Cost Prediction; Production Line Modeling, etc. The project manager should ensure that the appropriate tools are used at the right time and that the results are acted on.

XI. DOCUMENTATION

The development of any drug delivery device must be properly documented to satisfy regulatory authorities. Because the demands of regulators in different countries differ and demands are constantly developing, it is difficult to predict, with any certainty, what an individual case will require. Frequently, the decision about whether the device should follow the device or the drug route to regulatory approval is taken relatively late. Consequently, it is as well to start documenting properly as early as possible in the project. The device development has some additional areas of documentation required when compared with the development of a new chemical entity. For example, the discipline of configuration control should be applied early. This requires proper control of part drawings, assembly instructions, and so on. This aspect of developments is frequently slapdash resulting in confusion and unnecessary work during the development and regulatory embarrassment at the end.

XII. CONCLUSION

The most critical skill of the device development project manager is the ability to coordinate the activities of many skills in the three major skill groupings, of which two might be in an organization outside the project manager's own. To do this requires awareness of many disciplines, understanding device development thoroughly, and being a diplomat, planner, parent figure, and leader. A great deal can be delegated but the project manager cannot delegate responsibility for the overall project deliverables, for timeliness, for quality and for coordinating the functions.

The project manager has to speak the language of the formulation laboratory, the analytical laboratory, the focus group, the design suite, the tool room, and the workshop.

The project manager must use all the tools available effectively and ensure that the team do the same.

These skills are difficult to acquire. They come from training, experience, application, and a relentless attention to detail.

Underestimating the difficulty of device development leads, inevitably, to poor project management, delay, and failure.

Good device development management is worth a great deal by reducing time to market and improving the attractiveness of the complete product. It is worth investing in by giving it the appropriate priority and by training and developing the right people.

9

Clinical Trials—Quantum Leap or Last Gasp?
How Clinical Trials Can Make or Break a Drug Development Program

Leslie B. Rose

Medical Scientific Services Ltd.
Salisbury, England

The clinical phases of drug development present some of the most serious tests of management skills. The selected drug candidate demands rapidly escalating resources, in labor and cost, and, at the same time, much of the influence on progress is passed to third parties—the clinical investigators. The purpose of this chapter is to examine the special challenges encountered by the clinical project manager and to consider the skills and methods needed to bring successful medical products to market on time. It should be emphasized that these skills apply to all levels of clinical project management from the clinical development plan down to the individual trial and to project management at the strategic level.

I. ARE CLINICAL RESEARCH PROJECTS REALLY DIFFERENT?

A. Realism—Clinical Research's Holy Grail

There is a widespread management technique which imposes impossible goals with no expectation that they will be achieved. What the proponents of this method do expect is that another goal, secret and less demanding, will be achieved; the logic is that people will respond to unreasonable pressure by working harder than they would do if the target were realistic. You will not find this idea in any serious book about management because it does not work. People are demoralized by a continual sense of failure and do not respect unattainable objectives. Yet the author has worked for companies which practiced this and has many consultancy clients who are its victims.

This point is made to emphasize that the fundamentals of good project management are dealing openly with people on a realistic basis. In clinical trials, there are special reasons for adhering to these principles. Figure 1 gives some idea of the different people and disciplines with which the clinical research specialist has to interact. This illustration is not intended to show reporting lines or authority; the connections show the negotiations

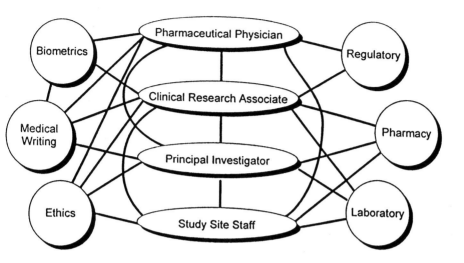

FIG. 1   Clinical research negotiations: Example of potential complexity.

which have to be carried out during the planning process and later when the study or program of studies is under way. The figure also shows the potential complexity of these negotiations and the high probability of failure unless a clear structure is implemented.

1. The Multidisciplinary Team

Some comment on the conventional team structure in clinical research is appropriate at this stage. Traditionally, the pharmaceutical physician has wielded most of the authority, but today this is all changing. A clear career structure is now available to nonmedical clinical scientists, so decision making will often be in the hands of experienced people whose qualifications do not necessarily include a medical degree. The main benefit of this trend is that a wider range of skills is available for managing clinical projects. Physicians are still necessary, but, now, they are members of multidisciplinary teams. In the traditional structure, both the pharmaceutical physician and the clinical research associate (CRA) have to negotiate with the study-site personnel, usually starting with the clinician who has overall authority for the site. Other study-site personnel may include research nurses, study-site coordinators, technicians, junior medical staff, and administrative staff (e.g., medical secretaries). Other disciplines within or connected to the site's institution may include pharmacists, laboratory staff, and ethics commit-tees. The purpose of this outline is not to itemize, exhaustively, all the dif-ferent people involved (the reader will already know these) but to highlight the potential complexity of the negotiations required. This complexity is a key feature of clinical trial projects and one in which they differ from re-search and development in many other industries. Exacerbating this com-plexity is the minimal control the project manager has over some external areas, such as patient recruitment or ethics committee approval.

2. The Customer or Client

One key person not shown in Fig. 1 is the internal client. Many companies are now operating a customer-oriented culture, which helps to clarify for whom any work is being done. Project management starts with the cus-tomer/client, who issues an initial requirement, and it is vital to be clear as to who this is. For a registration package of studies, the client could be the regulatory department, but might it not also be the marketing department, which will have to use the data? Other potential clients are the regulatory authorities, who issue specifications as to how the data should be submitted, the investigators who will be using the drug, and let us not forget the pa-tients! Thus, the more we look, the more complex the situation appears, with great potential for communication breakdown and project failure. Later in this chapter, we will look at ways of managing this web of different skills, interests (and possibly even objectives).

Contract research organizations (CROs) have some advantages be-cause they are usually clear as to who their client is. This is not because it is always obvious from the start, but they have to get it clear, or any nego-tiation is useless. The problems really occur when it is found later that the apparent client lacks the authority for key decisions. So careful review of plans and especially decision points is needed, and the correct responsibility must be assigned to each stage.

3. Modeling Reality in Project Planning

So, how can we plan realistically? How can we rely on the information we obtain from all of these people and build it into an effective plan? Let us start with the client, who issues the requirements for the clinical trial(s), and uses the results. If requirements were always clear to everyone, plan-ning would be far easier than it often is, but to a great extent, the time-hon-ored methodology for protocol development does not always give good re-sults. Consider Fig. 2, which shows a typical flow chart, distilled from various companies' standard operating procedures (SOPs). What, for ex-

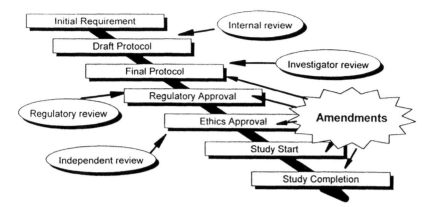

Typically 80% of protocols have amendments

FIG. 2 Protocol construction and progress: Conventional process.

ample, happens if the initial requirement is incomplete? Can we assume, safely, that the client has (a) thought of everything needed, and (b) has effectively communicated these needs in the requirement? Yet the conventional process makes just this assumption, with the result that gaps can remain unfilled or, perhaps, even worse, be filled erroneously by people further down the chain.

A second common problem with protocols is lack of focus on functional objectives. For example, a clear objective would be "To enable a decision on which patient population to target in the marketing campaign." A less clear objective would be "To evaluate the safety and efficacy of . . . ." The first offers a clear benefit from a successful trial, the second does not. If the drug turns out to be safe and effective (and we need criteria here), what are we going to do with the knowledge? This exemplifies the need for clear thinking and structured communication, usually with a wide range of people directly or indirectly involved in the trial. The author has encountered studies which started off with laudably clear objectives, but were published with very vague ones, presumably reflecting the quality of the data collected!

4. Study Designs and Methods

A common pitfall is insufficiently rigorous evaluation of study designs and methods. A "straw poll" during a clinical project management training course revealed that virtually all protocols have at least one amendment during the study. The reasons appear to cover the full range, from reliance on well-established designs without allowing newer, more creative ideas to be considered and, at the other extreme, not testing new methods for the current application. For example, in a recent angina study, treadmill exercise testing was used as the primary efficacy criterion. This is, of course, extremely well-validated methodology, but, in this case, the patients were elderly, so the exercise protocol was substantially modified to reduce the physical demand. The problem was that with such a mild exercise protocol, less than half the patients recruited showed sufficient electrocardiogram (ECG) changes to qualify for randomization. A quick pilot study would have alerted the sponsors before committing to major cost.

B. The Role of Senior Management

A recurring theme in clinical research is the role of senior management. By this we mean not the head of clinical research, not the head of R & D, but corporate management. The costs and risks of failure in the clinical phases are so large that they should be occupying much of top management's attention. Yet, in many companies, requirements, objectives, budgets, and deadlines, are imposed without any negotiation. On top of this, major changes are commonly dictated by management, usually by changing priorities. How can the clinical project manager fulfill top management's aspirations, within an increasingly constrained environment?

C. Predicting the Unpredictable—Managing Risk

All research and development must involve some risk. Figure 3 shows some of the risks typically encountered in the main stages of a typical clinical trial. The values for risk level and lateness are those usually applied in the author's company when planning studies. They may differ from those of the reader but are useful rules of thumb. Whatever rules are used, they will almost certainly be better than no risk assessment at all.

1. Risk Distribution in Clinical Phases

Delivering the results on time, to the required standard, may have a lower risk in phase I than in later phases, mainly because subjects are healthy and not potentially complicated patients, and thus, recruitment can be predicted with some confidence. However, first administration to humans is something of a leap into the unknown, and safety problems are always to

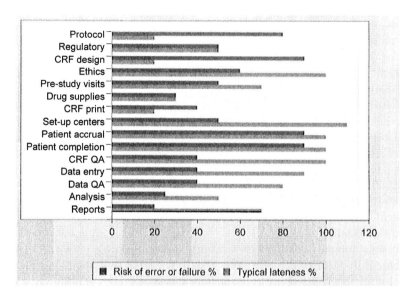

FIG. 3   Clinical research risks: Risk of error or failure and typical lateness.

be considered. What is possibly less obvious is the risk of any early-phase design errors to later phases and to the whole drug project.

Once phase III is imminent, perhaps there is a degree of confidence emerging, as much more is known about the drug. The requirement for phase III, therefore, may be seen as accumulating data to enable a product license application. In fact, the great expansion of activity dictated by phase III studies introduces even more complexity and a new set of risks. The application of the drug to a more realistic clinical setting means that we will not necessarily by studying "clean" patients. Patients will often have other diseases on top of that under study and will only be under observation for a small proportion of the time. Attention to protocol design, thus, is at least as critical as in phases I–II.

2. Key Tasks and External Agencies

The most common reason for late tasks and projects is that they started late. Before patients can be screened for entry, a well-established set of start-up tasks must be completed, and of these, some are relatively easy to plan, and others are less predictable. Those relying on internal agreements (e.g., drug supplies, protocol sign-off), can be expedited by instilling the right culture of negotiation between departments and individuals. But what of the external elements, particularly regulatory and ethics approvals? The former is, fortunately, reasonably easy to plan, because, in most countries, there are clear limits to the time and effort required to meet the regulators' requirements. Much more difficult is the matter of ethics approval. Across the European Union, ethics committee practices vary enormously, so that, when planning a multinational study, good local knowledge is essential. Even within the U.K. there is little consistency, especially since the demise of single central approval for multicenter studies. Theoretically, local research ethics committees (LRECs) are expected to follow Department of Health guidelines [1], but, if they choose not to do so, there is apparently no redress, so one may be presented with unexpected delays in particular centers because of widely varying LREC practices. There is a move towards rationalization in the U.K. in the form of a two-level approval process. A central committee will review the study and, if approved, pass it on to local committees for ratification. This has already been tried in at least one region in the U.K. with the result that it took up to six months to obtain approval because each LREC insisted on full review instead of ratification. Perhaps, here we have something to learn from the U.S., where the LREC equivalent, the Institutional Review Board (IRB) has clearer responsibilities and reporting lines and such delays are less common. In Australia, central approval is still possible, and the ethics committee sees itself as a more of a partner in research rather than a regulator, and very rapid study startup is possible.

The message here is that, if you do not have compelling reasons to conduct your studies in any particular country, be creative with your planning, and consider the big advantages you might gain in another part of the world. One European multinational does more clinical research in Australia than in any country outside its home base. If you are forced to live with the problems outlined above, obtain the best and most recent information you can from the LRECs and from their users, and build this realistically into your plans. The plans might not look as good as you would like, but you will have a better chance of keeping to them.

D. Quantity, Quality, Timeliness

Any discussion of clinical research planning and conduct sooner or later gravitates to the question of patient recruitment. The clinical version of Murphy's law states that as soon as you start a study, all the patients with that disease disappear! How realistically one can plan for recruitment depends very much on the type of study. For a stable chronic disease, such as essential hypertension, large volumes of data should be available to provide good estimates of the number of patients expected. This will come from medical practitioners' records, but it is vital to modify any estimating database for the current study. What the investigator observes is not that all the hypertensives disappear—there are just as many as ever—but that he had not applied the selection criteria when estimating recruitment. One of the author's client companies applies a standard 40 percent factor to all investigator recruitment estimates (i.e., they expect investigators to recruit 40 percent of what they predict). This is seldom completely accurate for an individual center (although much better than the original estimate), but averages quite well across all the centers.

More sophisticated approaches to recruitment statistics are being evaluated. These data can be converted into valuable metrics for selecting sites (rather than for monitoring progress), especially if they are reduced to an ordinal scale [2], thus, making comparisons between sites simpler. The values can be adjusted for other factors, such as the proportion of patients evaluable, the monitor time spent on-site (a reflection of data quality), and the number of data queries, to give a global measure of site performance.

For acute diseases, there is a higher risk that recruitment estimates are inaccurate because one is assuming that new cases arise with predictable frequency. For instance, some conditions are strongly seasonal, and some seasons will be better (or worse) than others. So it is vital to retrieve data far back enough in time to avoid being misled by an unusually high-prevalence season. Even if we are reassured by this, we should still ask the all-important project manager's question What happens if . . . ? In this case, What happens if the next season is unusually benign?

1. Protocol Compliance

Earlier, we considered the challenge of achieving a protocol which does not need to be amended. Even if we meet this challenge, the next one is to ensure compliance. If the protocol is difficult to follow, and even if we have no problems in finding patients (a rare scenario), there is still the great danger that many of these patients are invalidated by protocol violations because the drug is now being used in the real world of clinical medicine. If it is critical that clinic assessments are carried out at particular times of day (for example, to coincide with trough drug levels or to plot the time course of postdose response), how confident can we be that this will be observed? Can we measure the impact on the study of exceptions to the rule? Can we estimate how many valid patients we might lose?

2. The Data Cleaning Cycle

We may not only lose data because of protocol violations. Quality of work varies widely between centers, so what contingency should we include to allow for query resolution and consequent delays to database lock? With most companies maintaining records of investigator performance, this is critical information to include. If queries are being tracked electronically, it is relatively simple to generate statistics on data query incidence and turnaround. However, these are traditionally used mainly to feed performance data back to centers during the study, rather than for planning new projects. Detailed information on study center quality performance is a powerful planning tool [2]. The author's company has excluded some high-recruiting centers from new studies because protocol compliance and data quality are so poor that many patients recruited are invalid. Interestingly, there is no evidence that so-called centers of excellence, the high-profile teaching hospital units, are any better in this regard, and their quality performance is usually inferior to a well-trained general practice center.

E. Clinical Trial Risk Management—A Summary

Clearly, any detailed examination of clinical trial risks could fill a whole chapter, and here we have discussed just some of those which have been prominent in the author's experience. No doubt, this section has raised more questions than answers, and this, indeed, is the essence of the message. Unless the project manager asks those questions, based on "What happens if . . . ?," the most elegant plans will be vulnerable to sudden and unexpected change or will be destroyed altogether. Perhaps this is why 90 percent of project management software purchasers just use it to do initial planning and never update their plans—it would be too disappointing if they did!

F. Getting More from Less—Multiple Projects, Priorities, Workload, Progress Control

All of the complexity described so far would apply even if each person were involved with only one clinical trial. The reality is that most people are doing all of this for several trials, multiplying the problems and introducing new ones. This is substantially different from where project management grew up, in construction and engineering. The generally accepted view there is of a manager responsible for one project, although this may be anything from the local apartment block to the Channel Tunnel. Thus, clinical research is in the forefront of developing new project management approaches in a high-risk industry.

1. The Need for Policies on Prioritization

To get some sense out of conflicting multiple clinical trials, some form of prioritization is necessary, and it helps to reduce this to as simple a level as possible. One company was accustomed to assigning individual priority levels to all of its clinical trials, so that there might be as many as 40 levels. The problem was that no one could remember the actual priority of each study, so, levels were not adhered to and were open to change without notice by senior management. Because so many other factors can influence the sequencing of trials, holding some up and releasing others, it is perfectly possible to manage them with as few as three priority levels (although some of the software systems confusingly allow many levels).

2. Priority or Urgency?

In recent years conferences on crisis management have been increasingly popular. Although much of the focus has been on drug safety crises, nevertheless, the great interest in the concept shows how much we tend to enjoy an emergency—team spirit is always high, and there is a great sense of achievement at the end. But often the problem is not a genuinely unforeseeable one arising externally but simply a conflict of priorities. Figure 4 shows one clinical trial which is running late, and another trial is scheduled to start immediately after staff are available from completing the first. What usually happens is that the second project is delayed because of the need to finish the first, and this then feeds through the whole program until all of the projects are late and, thus, managed as crises. A better technique is to recognize the high priority of trial 1 at the outset and do everything possible to complete it on time, even if this means extra staff or other expense. Then, this breaks the vicious circle of crisis feeding crisis. An additional benefit is that, if projects are scheduled sequentially rather than in parallel, total investment is less and profitability is higher. This works in the following way. Figure 5 shows that, if two projects are conducted at once, there can be no return on investment until they are both completed. If one project is held up, and twice the effort put into the other, cash flow starts earlier, maximum investment is less (because the first helps to pay for the second), yet the second project is no later in completing. To put this into a clinical trial perspective, should you try to run two phase III anti-infectives programs at the same time? You might do better to put all your skilled people and budget on one of them, run twice as many study centers, and finish it

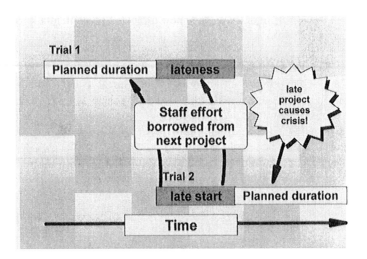

FIG. 4 Priority problems: Why unstable priority levels generate repeated crises. Courtesy of A. E. Berridge, Technical Management Development Ltd. (adapted).

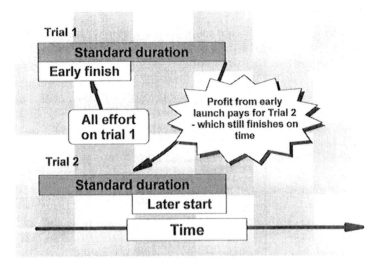

FIG. 5 Trials in parallel or series? Courtesy of A. E. Berridge, Technical Management Development Ltd. (adapted).

earlier. An early launch will win you more patent protection and get in front of more of your competitors. The second program will be no later than if you had run them at the same time.

Admittedly the clinical project manager rarely has the freedom to make such decisions and, instead, has to manage conflicting resource demands by developing his/her own rules for deciding priorities. The answer to give when a new project is imposed by top management is not "No," but "Yes—but we can't start until . . . ."

G. Progress Information—Can We Believe It?

If you have read this far, you will see that project management software can be far more than just a planning tool. You can be updating your plans to give you ongoing control of your clinical trials (although it has been said that software does not manage projects, only people do). To do this, reliable information on study progress is needed, and the word "reliable" is vital. The most commonly-used measure is patient recruitment, but this is only of value if it is clearly defined. Do we mean number of patients screened, number randomized, number valid for efficacy analysis, or any of a host of other definitions? Unless these definitions are clear from the outset, progress will be impossible to control properly. The best way to define progress points is by using items which can be proven ("deliverables")—Is there physical evidence of the clean case report forms (CRFs) in-house, for example? Unproven information may still be useful for giving early warning of problems but should not be relied upon for reporting progress to senior management.

H. Senior Management Revisited

Reports to management tend to consume huge amounts of effort. One country affiliate is required to send a clinical research report to its overseas head office, and this report runs to at least 80 pages every month. Much of the information is repeated from previous months, and all the multitude of details cannot be read by all the recipients—they would never have the time. The key to effective reporting lies with the project manager, who must get agreement on what information is necessary and when. Much the same applies to progress meetings, which are usually used to report progress. If concise, easily understood reports have already been issued, why repeat the exercise during the meeting? It is far better to use the time for decisions based on information already available, so here is another role for the project manager, catalyzing effective meetings.

I. Multidisciplinary Teamworking

Earlier we emphasized the multidisciplinary nature of modern drug development. So diverse are the skills required, that understanding between the skill holders may be incomplete. Therefore, the project manager must be a generalist, appreciating (but not necessarily understanding in-depth) a wide range of technical issues. This begs the question of who is really in charge. As we have already seen, transfer of data from one stage to the next is less successful if the authority is transferred abruptly at the same time—continuity is essential. One approach, used in passing manufacturing methods from phase I onward, is to involve the later phase specialists as observers and advisers in the early-phase teams, and vice versa. However the key lies in lines of authority—to whom should the project managers report? It will be argued here that they should report to top management. If they report to anyone else, how can their authority be real?

II. A NEW WORLD OF CLINICAL RESEARCH

A. Projects versus Hierarchies—New Solutions

The most desirable type of project organization and simplest to implement is the self-contained project, which can be treated almost as a separate company. However, this can be justified only if the team members are spending most of the time on the one project. More realistically, people are shared between projects, and then, it makes sense for people to be allocated to project teams by agreement with their functional heads. These agreements need to be clear, usually in writing, and once agreed, the functional head must not override it. Therefore, a key function of the project manager is to negotiate these agreements and ensure that top management supports compliance with them. A somewhat looser structure is also possible, where staff are simply "rented" from departments and allocated to projects, as many companies use contracted-in staff. Whatever the structure, how the staff time is paid for needs to be agreed on, but in practice this is rarely monitored in pharmaceutical development so that the real cost of an individual project is difficult to measure. This is the reason that CRO work sometimes looks expensive.

1. Who Is the New Clinical Project Manager?

There is a welcome trend in pharmaceuticals toward a flatter management structure, with the project teams receiving more prominence than fixed hierarchies. Nevertheless, departmental heads generally have more status and benefits than project managers, and the latter, if successful, may be offered promotion to run a department. Here, we will suggest an alternative view because clinical projects are challenging and require very special skills. In fact, they are so demanding that successfully completing clinical projects on time may be more difficult than running a department! The scenario of a departmental head being promoted to project manager is not to be discounted.

2. Candidates for Project Responsibility

Although much progress is being made, the true definition of the project manager's role is still emerging. Projects may be managed by people holding the titles of pharmaceutical physician, clinical research associate, project coordinator, clinical trials manager, among many others. Conversely, some project managers do not actually manage projects, but may only provide services to people who do. Whatever the title, the same skills and functions will be involved, but there is the danger that project responsibility will be thrust upon individuals without the right training or experience or without the authority required to get things done.

In this context, perhaps the most difficult of the roles outlined above is the project coordinator. As this implies, this individual has to do all the work of negotiating plans, but has none of the authority to ensure compliance with plans. It is a very common management structure, and, in most applications, usually the worst structure to choose. It can be made to work, but only if the coordinator receives authoritative backup from elsewhere—otherwise, what is the point of good planning if people can default on agreements without sanctions?

3. Approaches to Project Organization

Some companies are responding creatively to these challenges by implementing more rational organizational structures. For example, it is recognized that people who have prolific ideas are generally less effective at executing them. An approach being tried now with some success is to accept that it is difficult to change a person's fundamental nature, so the clinical research function is divided into two groups. One group generates ideas and refines them into workable projects, and then, these are passed to the other group with the skills to carry out the projects. The danger lies in effective transfer of the project from one group to the other—indeed this applies at many stages throughout the R & D process. Therefore, the team members who execute the plan must be involved in its design. A similar problem can occur when a drug moves between clinical phases. For instance, unless the phase II specialists are involved in agreeing to and accepting the phase I results, at least two problems might occur. First, the phase I results might not meet the requirements to enter phase II, and secondly, the phase II specialists might not accept the results even if correct. This highlights the need for open and regular communication and involvement of people on a team basis.

4. Project Manager Functions

It may appear to the reader that the clinical project manager is almost a mythical beast, requiring amazing personal and professional attributes. Figure 6 shows the main functions to be fulfilled. Compare this with Fig. 1. What is different is that the complexity has been reduced by breaking it down into logical stages, each stage having clear channels of communication. Scientists are usually very good at managing such a structure, because of their analytical approach to planning (and problems). This is more a valuable by-product of being a scientist, than the main reason for the qualification, which is to know enough to assess that what one is being told is true—vital at the planning stages. However, it is hardly practical to engage a technical specialist to manage every new project, and, indeed, it is not

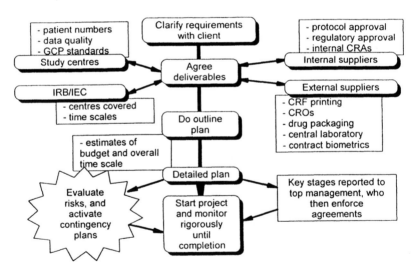

FIG. 6   Project Manager Functions. Courtesy of A. E. Berridge, Technical Management Development Ltd. (adapted).

necessary. Some companies (more commonly smaller start-up ones) pride themselves in employing only Ph.D.s and postgraduate-qualified physicians to run clinical trials. This reflects the specialist nature of these companies, but, as they develop, they usually take on new projects outside their original technical specialties. Are they going to replace all the project staff as they do this? In fact, they manage very well with their existing people, who turn out to be more adaptable than they thought. Thus, very many Ph.D.s in pharmaceutical clinical development are working outside the subjects of their theses. It should be understood here that we are discussing the project management role—there will of course always be a need for specialists within multidisciplinary project teams, and such specialists commonly become project managers in their own right because of their management skills rather than technical expertise.

These skills include the ability to take in a situation in breadth, looking for interfaces between seemingly unconnected issues. This, coupled with tenacity under stress, builds a culture of forward-looking management—predicting problems, minimizing the need to find scapegoats, and always working toward attaining the project targets on time. Interpersonal skills are also vital, and these come into play at every stage from project design, when agreements between various disciplines have to be negotiated, to the collection of accurate progress information.

B. Consistent Planning

The structure for protocol development shown at the beginning of this chapter is typical of procedures commonly used in the pharmaceutical industry. It complies with good clinical practice (GCP), and, assuming all the correct data are passed down the line, would be expected to generate a workable protocol. This is not always the case because of its unidirectional design. A list of requirements at the outset is unlikely to be complete, and, unless this list is challenged by the recipient, gaps may remain unfilled, or even worse, may be filled by guesswork. A more secure system is shown in Fig. 7, which is successfully used by the author for all types of work related to clinical trials. The essence is that at the functional requirements stage (what the client wants from the project) and at the selection of methodology stage, two-way communication with the client is the rule. Tools which help this process are already largely available in the form of SOPs to check feasibility and databases of information on how methods performed in the past, to name but two. A project manager with a good grasp of this process should be able to define any project within his span of technical knowledge,

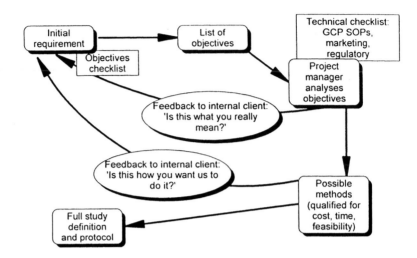

FIG. 7   Protocol definition: Alternative process. Courtesy of A. E. Berridge, Technical Management Development Ltd. (adapted).

as long as he is empowered by top management to carry out the negotiations required. Projects too often fail when this empowerment has not been carried out (such as the project coordinator).

Precisely the same process can be used at any level in clinical research, whether one is planning a single study or a whole clinical development program. In practice within pharmaceutical companies, the latter more often resembles Fig. 2, probably because, at this stage, much less is clear about the whole drug project. For single studies, the trap to avoid is using tried and tested methods on a production line basis. This can stifle creativity.

C. New Approaches to Written Procedures

Standard operating procedures (SOPs) have come a very long way since GCP entered common parlance over ten years ago. We are now seeing graphical representations of familiar processes, which aid understanding and compliance. We have already seen how SOPs provide essential tools at the project design stage, as they include standard checklists against which objectives and methods can be measured. Although clinical trials would stagnate without trying innovative methods, some standardization is a valuable time saver—if this were not so, our operating procedures would not be

For each task -

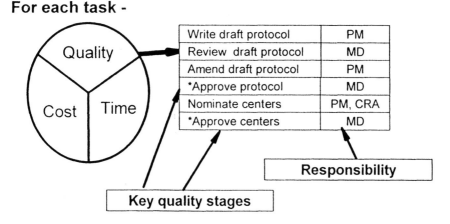

Write draft protocol	PM
Review draft protocol	MD
Amend draft protocol	PM
*Approve protocol	MD
Nominate centers	PM, CRA
*Approve centers	MD

Responsibility

Key quality stages

FIG. 8   Extract from clinical project template.

standard. The same applies to clinical project plans, so if we have standardized our practices we will be using common project structures for similar studies. Figure 8 shows part of a typical task list, which could apply with modification to a wide range of clinical trials and which can be included in an SOP as a template. Resources and duration for each task can be estimated for each new project, which can rapidly generate budgets and overall timescales. If the SOP is followed, this means that alternative studies, or those competing for resources, are directly comparable.

D. The Quality Dimension

As well as the highly structured world of GCP, which is benefiting from project management, we are now seeing the influence of a third management philosophy. Quality systems are not at all new. The modern, internationally recognized standard ISO 9000 has its roots in military equipment supply in the 1950s, and has progressed via BS 5750 in the United Kingdom [3]. In addition, the term "total quality management" is widely used (although not universally defined). Whatever quality system is being used, it is far more effective if it is integrated with existing management structures, rather than imposed as another layer. In the author's company, a contract research organization, two main actions have been taken to achieve this. First, all procedures have been restructured to comply with ISO 9000 and with the existing project management system. Second, key quality steps are included in each clinical project plan, as shown in Fig. 8. Thus, the project management system ensures compliance with the quality and the GCP requirements of the study. In addition, with the study's critical path clearly highlighted, we are alerted to the tasks which must achieve quality approval first time, or they will delay the whole project.

E. Integrating GCP, Quality Systems, and Project Management

But as we have seen, one of the project manager's needs is to cope with new challenges from new project ideas. So it is not possible to standardize everything. Several pharmaceutical companies and CROs have approached this with procedures at several levels. Figure 9 shows one such approach. The more familiar SOPs contain completely standard material, with the project templates discussed above. At the working level, the varying requirements of individual studies can be accommodated with work procedures, which contain only material specific to that study, especially where a departure from standard practice is necessary. The baseline project plan for the study will be included as an appendix.

In between, other documents may be needed. For example, if the organization has any areas of specialization, a procedure for that special process may be written. Finally, governing all operations and projects are the quality manual and quality procedures, the first of which states policy and the second sets out methods for ensuring that quality policy is met.

One word of warning on quality systems: They are of no use unless they actually improve business performance. A recent survey [4] suggests that a

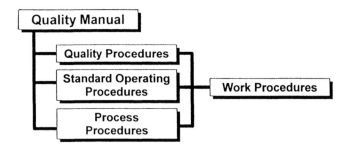

FIG. 9   Procedures for quality: As implemented in a contract research organization.

majority of companies across all industries have not achieved the expected business benefits from implementing ISO 9000. They are mostly forced to implement it because it was expected by their customers. Management must have clear objectives as to the improvements sought and the means to monitor these improvements, rather than using any quality system just for public relations or enhancing credibility.

1. Procedures for Projects

There is one further SOP which does not seem to appear in any pharmaceutical company's register. This should cover project management methods. Examples of its content would be how project managers are appointed, how their authority (or empowerment) is defined, their responsibilities, the stages of setting up and running a clinical trial project—in fact, all the areas discussed in this chapter and many more.

Many companies will have such a document for running drug projects at the strategic level—indeed, this is the level at which the discipline is most advanced. However, it will be more difficult to achieve top level objectives if individual smaller projects, clinical trials and many others, are not managed effectively at the operational level. Thus, the clinical project manager has the tough job of ensuring good communication with other levels of management. It is hardly practical for strategic project managers to track all the tasks in every individual project, so agreement has to be achieved as to which key stages will provide the interface links to enable effective whole drug project tracking. Suitable stages would be best defined as deliverables, such as the approved protocol for a pivotal phase III trial or its final report.

F. Getting Things Done—The Clinical Project Manager's Authority

At several stages in this chapter, the project manager's vital need for top management support has been emphasized. If this one need were satisfied, many companies which are now average performers, would be among the leaders in their fields. This is graphically illustrated by a survey carried out in 1994 [5]. Fifty chief executives from U.K. pharmaceutical companies were approached by letter to participate. The subject was top management's attitudes toward critical issues in delivering clinical trial results on time. In return for a brief interview, the participants were offered free consultancy to assess their current clinical project systems and to suggest changes. What is significant about the survey is not how many responded (four), but that the vast majority immediately delegated the matter to their clinical research people (who did not respond). The clear message was that most chief executives are not worrying at all about meeting clinical research objectives and see it as their subordinates' problem. This could be understood if it applied to drug discovery or preclinical research, but clinical trials are consuming resources and timescales at an escalating rate. If the really worrying issues get such scant attention, is it surprising that project managers lack support? It may well be argued that managers should be empowering staff by delegation, but there is a big difference between offloading responsibility wholesale and delegating key decisions which are backed up by the authority to get them enacted.

G. How to Create Empowerment

Even if one's own scenario seems so disappointing, there is hope! If many of the causes of project failure are related to poor communications, the project manager can achieve much by ensuring that what has been agreed to is widely known within the organization, especially in the upper strata. When a clinical plan or protocol has been agreed upon, why not send a summary to top management, itemizing the key deliverables, who is responsible, and when they have been promised. Even if top management does nothing, is it more or less likely that drug supply (for example) will be on time and correctly packaged, when pharmacy department knows who is aware of the agreement? Eventually, of course, top management starts to take some notice of these succinct summaries from clinical research, especially when they are followed by positive progress reports.

H. Clinical Research in the New Global Village

As long as pharmaceuticals continue to be produced, clinical trials will be necessary. Among the many questions are Who can afford to do them, where will they be done, and how will possible changes in practice affect their management?

Many factors are influencing the world of clinical research, and we will speculate on just two. The first is impossible to ignore, and that is the headlong development of information technology, which impacts on most areas of business and daily life. To begin at the beginning, there is enormous scope for improving the planning stages of clinical trials, especially in collecting information to produce estimates of timescale, cost, and labor. Looking first at cost, an initiative is already in place with the PICAS™ database [6]. This attempts to compare investigational site costs. The data source is costs from actual studies carried out by subscribing companies.

This database will probably take several years to settle down, but it is one of the first attempts to base cost estimates on real data from across the industry. Some companies are already learning to apply their own correction factors to PICAS™ data.

1. Cracking the Patient Supply Problem

Probably the most critical estimate needed is the rate of patient accrual, and here there is the opportunity for substantial progress. Some clinical study sites are beginning to organize their patient records far more effectively. This is a trend starting in the U.S. [7], with organizations offering databases of patients who can be matched to protocol selection criteria. The patients can be contacted directly and screening clinic visits scheduled very quickly. Such advertising may raise questions in Europe, but whatever the ethics, this shows how technology can change what has been traditionally the clinical research manager's nightmare—finding enough valid patients.

2. The Cautious Approach

The availability of such volumes of data enables more widespread application of a hugely underused method, the feasibility study or pilot study. The former is really a paper (now electronic) exercise, where we can simulate the clinical trial [8] before committing to major cost. Previously, such studies have been of limited value because the data source was unreliable or nonexistent, but now the world is changing. Interestingly, the concept may be more easily applied in general practice than in hospital medicine, because of the widespread use of computerized patient records in the former (at least in much of Europe). In the U.K., hospital patient records are mostly paper, and commonly fragmented and disparate. Only in dedicated clinical research units does one find a serious attempt at organizing patient records for ready access. There is, though, a basis for optimism, with U.K. hospital trusts now processing data on admissions, referrals, and outcomes, mainly for marketing reasons. Reasons for referral are coded using much the same dictionaries as are used by the drug industry in biometrics. So it is not too much of an extrapolation to see such codes helping to identify patients eligible for a particular study. However, this presupposes a fundamental change in the role of research among health care providers, of which more a little later. An interim approach may be to issue cheap pocket computers to clinicians, into which they can enter basic patient information during each consultation. Quality assurance of such data may be difficult but should provide much better guidance on referral rates than is generally available at present.

3. Automating Progress Control

Because of the need to integrate diverse disciplines in clinical trials, any tool which can improve communications is of immense value. Thus, various forms of remote data collection are being evaluated, even using the Internet. Although the impetus of this comes from the need to speed data collection, there may be a valuable by-product for the project manager. If one of the most difficult tasks is to collect reliable progress data from study centers, it is going to be much easier if the manager is physically linked with the center and can actually see the data which prove the progress claimed. This could form the first link in an almost fully automated progress control system, as shown in Fig. 10.

All progress control systems need to collect data on achievement of objectives (time and deliverables), and costs, which will be actual cash and work time expended. The diagram is not exhaustive and gives examples of sources of automated progress data. As many of the deliverables are documents, and if there is a document management system which tracks key stages (protocol sign-off, for instance), then, these stages might be linked directly with the project planning system, updating the plan immediately as the deliverable is proven. Similarly, cost information could come via an electronic link with the company's accounting system, which would use unique cost codes for particular clinical trial activities. As speculated above, direct data accrual could feed patient progress information straight into the

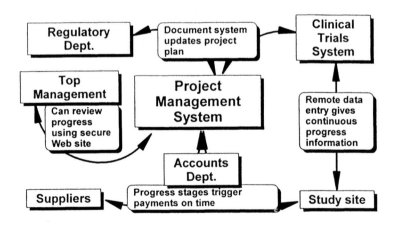

FIG. 10   Study management: New possibilities for automation.

project planning system. In addition, all of the office-based work can be automatically tracked, even with current technology. With virtually everyone using a computer, a memory resident program can monitor time spent on individual tasks, for which the user must identify the task worked on. Future technology would be intelligent enough to identify the task itself. This still leaves some tasks, such as site visits, to be reported manually. However, even this could eventually be automated to a large extent because monitoring reports today are commonly completed on-site on a portable computer for later upload to the central office, and this could track the time spent on-site.

The great benefit of these possibilities is that it will relieve the project manager of much of the work of collecting the information and checking its validity. Yes, such semi-intelligent systems will make a few guesses about what is actually happening at any one time, but it is very much the author's experience that approximate progress data is far better than none at all (or perhaps worse, data which are later found to be invalid). The team members will also be delighted because they will not have to fill in any more time sheets!

Would such a system find ready acceptance among clinical research specialists? It is possible that they might regard it as a policing system, but if trials are being seriously carried out as professionally managed projects, such data will already be collected conventionally. Only the manner of collection will have changed. If people really are worried about task time data being picked up automatically, were they reporting it accurately before?

What can be done with the current state of the art? Some form of computerized clinical trial management system is now commonplace, although the data are usually entered manually. What generally happens is that reports are generated by such a system at intervals, and these are used to reenter progress information into the project planning system. Although there does not appear to be a fully integrated trial management and project planning system available off the shelf, computer linkage is possible, which eliminates transcription errors and keeps the project plan more up to date.

4. Building Tighter Teams

The second area of crystal ball gazing is closely related to the first, as the IT revolution makes so many things possible. At the very beginning of the chapter, we looked at the disparate interests of the people involved in a typical study and the way they are conventionally managed. It is our view that there will be a move toward bringing clinical investigators much closer to the inner project team. At present they are hardly regarded as team

members at all, but much rather as suppliers contracted to deliver valid
patients (or conversely, customers who need to be influenced). Almost in-
stant communications are already bringing people into close and regular
contact, often without ever meeting, and it is amazingly quick and easy (and
inexpensive) to send an E-mail message anywhere in the world. This will
never obviate the need for site visits (you have to go there to see for yourself), but, in between such visits, contacts can be far more frequent. Those
with any experience as clinical research associates will understand the frustration of trying to contact a busy consultant by telephone, but with E-mail
the parties do not have to talk in real time—their mail is waiting to be read
whenever they are ready. A sense of involvement will be far more easily
achieved with a dedicated (and secure) Internet web site for the study,
which can contain the very latest information and can be interactive.

What we are creating here is a kind of virtual team territory, which the
project can call its own. For projects carried out entirely on one geographical site, a physical meeting place is a traditional team building method, but,
for multicenter and multinational clinical projects, we have had to make do
with regional meetings held fairly infrequently because of cost and time
constraints. Video conferencing may have a place, but the cost and compli-
cation are still high. Although Internet technology does not yet have the
capacity to make real-time video practical, cheap text- and voice-based conferencing are already here—and you can exchange graphics and video clips
while you talk.

In Fig. 11, the study site is shown as one of the external elements with
which the project team has to interact—not even one of the outer (part-
time) team members. Surely performance is going to be far better if study
sites can be brought much closer to the inner team. With virtual team territory, we may be a step nearer this goal.

5. Changing Attitudes in Health Care

In most developed countries, the current major changes in providing health
care involve a more market-oriented model. Hospitals and primary care
organizations are extending their market concept to include clinical trials
as a source of extra revenue. Again, the New World nations have grasped
the initiative, and we have already discussed here how the clinical function
can organize itself to provide much better value to those commissioning
clinical research. In the U.K., the National Health Service is breaking out
of its institutional straightjacket, and a number of the new hospital trusts
are considering formal organizations and partnerships to manage their research activities. The NHS now has a national Director of Trials, indicating

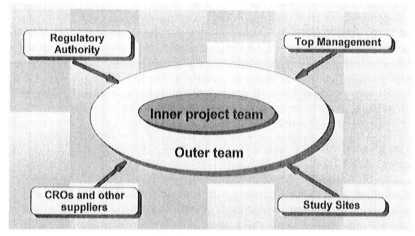

FIG. 11 Clinical project teams: Relationships between inner and outer teams and external groups. Courtesy of A. E. Berridge, Technical Management Development Ltd. (adapted).

that this is being taken seriously at a high level. But how can such a partnership make a really positive contribution?

6. Consolidating Agendas

The key is surely in the word partnership. At present, all parties value their independence highly and will oppose any apparent attempt to erode it. Consultants do not want to be told what studies they should be taking on, ethics committees must be free to consider each protocol without strings attached, and pharmacies will discourage any extension of the formulary, to name a few. Therefore, an integrated clinical trials function within a medical care facility, first, must clarify what the benefits will be for all potential partners and who are the potential beneficiaries. There can be no new drugs without clinical trials, so, the ultimate beneficiaries are the patients. Along the way, there will be others, such as saving money for health service by treating patients more quickly, the manufacturer sustaining its continued research from the new drug's profits, and of course the medical care facility receiving income from the trials it undertakes. This is looking at the situation positively. The converse is that, with the world rapidly becoming an electronic village, it matters less and less where one carries out one's research program. Indeed, the continuing International Conference on Harmonisation should ultimately mean that data for marketing authorizations will be in common formats worldwide and to common standards (although admittedly this goal is some way in the future). Medical communities which continue to adhere to a cottage industry mentality in clinical research may find themselves sidelined in favor of the better organized.

7. A Vision of the Future

Therefore, these well-organized centers will be taking on all the systems and methods familiar to the pharmaceutical companies: GCP, quality systems, and, of course, project management. The opportunity for the business community is there for the taking—to transfer these skills to the medical community while there is still time. One of the great strengths both of GCP and project management is the concept of accountability. GCP clearly states the obligations of the parties involved, and project management enables compliance by building the obligations into plans which can be carried out effectively. The major risks which we discussed earlier, among which clinical data volume and quality failures are very prominent, must be addressed by clinical centers.

It is not acceptable for principal investigators to sign protocols without reading them and to delegate all the work to junior staff who lack the proper training and time to meet the study's targets (and still to collect the fees). This may sound excessively negative, but it is commonplace in many active clinical research centers.

Formal quality systems are surely set to become more integrated into project plans, rather than a kind of afterthought ("oh yes, we must schedule a site audit some time"). This will take the form that deliverables become more accurately specified in plans, so that it is clearer when they have been achieved—and this will happen at all levels from the data source to the sponsor's top management. The clinical project manager must add to the classical triad for each task—technical objective, cost, and time delivered—the quality standard specified and how it will be proven.

More automation at study sites will enable far better estimates and, thus, more realistic plans, because valid data will be available. Health service data will become properly organized to enable "data mining" for feasibility studies, lessening the chances of embarking on unsound clinical trials.

With globalization rapidly overtaking drug development [9], all of these new tools will need to be adapted for use across different cultures. In practice, it will almost certainly not be possible to harmonize at the clinical site level to any useful extent, because medical practice is organized so differently around the world. Therefore, project management must pay even more attention to forging multilevel links between strategy and operations. National subprojects can tailor their management to local needs, and planning and progress control will consolidate project data at an appropriate level of detail. One useful approach in such a scenario is for the manager to plan only deliverables and to let project teams worry about how they will meet their objectives. Thus, the project plan becomes a list of deliverables (what do we have to produce?), not a list of tasks (what are we going to do?). Curiously, some project software pays scant attention to deliverables. The author recently evaluated a new software system which did not have the term in its database, and the help desk staff had never heard of it! The simple solution is to use the task field to enter the deliverable—it is really a matter of terminology, but the intellectual difference is important.

This focus on deliverables is a fitting note on which to conclude. So much effort can be wasted in pharmaceutical development by worrying about what we have to do, rather than what we should be handing over to the next stage. If this relatively simple attitude change could be achieved across all the disciplines in clinical research, the industry would have a much more secure future. Technology is now becoming available to communicate such a change to everyone involved, so there will be no excuse for not doing it. It will be much easier to achieve the clarity of purpose which is vital for survival into the next millennium, if the following key concepts can be incorporated into the drug development program:

* planning based on real data rather than guesswork and optimism,
* active participation in planning by multidisciplinary teams,
* empowerment of clinical project managers by top management, which will need clearer definitions of responsibility and authority, and
* bringing clinical study sites closer to the inner project team.

ACKNOWLEDGMENT

The author gratefully acknowledges the contribution of Tony Berridge, Director of Technical Management Development Ltd, and Non-Executive Director of Medical Scientific Services Ltd, for reading the manuscript, for helpful comments, and for permission to use material for some of the illustrations.

REFERENCES

1. Department of Health. Local Research Ethics Committees. *HMSO Dd DH 003009 7/92 C20 G3392 38776.*

2. L Kirby. Quantification at clinical sites. *Appl. Clin. Trials 5*: 11: 26–30, 1996.
3. British Standards Institute. *BS EN ISO 9002: 1994*: Quality Systems: Model for quality assurance in production, installation and servicing. 1994.
4. J Seddon. ISO 9000 implementation and value-added: Three case studies. *Report available from Vanguard Consulting Ltd*, via the author, 1996.
5. L B Rose. Top management attitudes to clinical research performance in the pharmaceutical industry. *Internal Report, Medical Scientific Services Ltd.*, 1994.
6. H Glass. How to get accurate information so that you can effectively benchmark your R & D success. Proceedings of IIR Ltd Conference on Measurement of Performance in Pharmaceutical R & D, October 1996. Reported in *Pharm. Physician 8*: 3: 27–34, 1996.
7. C Petersen. New strategies for academic medical centers. *Appl. Clin. Trials 5*: 8: 33–40, 1996.
8. M Hale, W R Gillespie, S K Gupta et al. Clinical trial simulation. *Appl. Clin. Trials 5*: 8: 35–40, 1996.
9. L Brown. ICH GCP and its worldwide implementation. *Good Clin. Pract. J. 3*: 4: 6–9, 1996.

10

Manufacturing Project Management

Stephen R. Self

Merck Generics Ltd.
Kent, England

I. INTRODUCTION

The pharmaceutical industry has faced a very changeable environment in the last ten years. A more competitive market which has been changed structurally by the influence of many more groups involved in purchasing decisions, has led to greater pressure on prices and profits. Complex development programs and the increasing costs of product development have forced all companies to examine the development process to improve efficiency, cost-effectiveness and shorten lead times. One area of significant improvement has been project management in product development. More attention is being paid to integrating R & D activities worldwide to reduce development times and improve the focus on commercial outcome. Improving the coordination of preclinical, clinical, and technical activities is now well in hand in most organizations, and great strides are being made in planning and executing development programs. In addition, it has been acknowledged that better integration of R & D and Marketing is needed to ensure that development targets areas of greatest commercial interest and scientific feasibility. R & D and Marketing have, therefore, worked more closely integrating their activities at portfolio and project level to optimize the chances of a stream of products which meet the company's financial objectives.

The improvement in the development process has undoubtedly been focused primarily on R & D and Marketing. Although this has strengthened product development considerably, it still falls short of a complete overhaul of the process to fully integrate all functions into the product development effort. An area that still needs to receive full attention is Manufacturing. The question is why? It could be argued that this has been caused by an attitudinal problem on both sides of the equation. In the past Manufacturing has essentially been seen and has seen itself as a reactive function which has to deal with the outcome of development but does not influence the process itself. In the past when prices and margins have been high, there was less incentive to examine the cost and manufacturability of the products throughout the development process. However, in the last ten years this approach has come under increasing challenge for a number of reasons. The main ones are the following:

As development programs are shortened, the scale-up of primary and secondary processes has to be more rapid to meet the demands of a large development program.

More process validation data are being demanded by authorities to demonstrate that there is a well-controlled and well-understood process. Nowhere is this more true than in the biotech field where the process and the product are essentially one and the same, and controls to demonstrate a reproducible and robust process are essential for eventual approval of the product. Preparation for the Preapproval Inspection at the site of manufacture also places more demands on the manufacturing team.

The need to reach peak sales worldwide much earlier in the product life cycle means a rapid growth of product supply and hence the need for a more robust process. Therefore, manufacturability must be "engineered in" rather than "bolted on." There is also a need for greater flexibility in the potential number of variants needed by the market to ensure that the molecule is maximally exploited during its short patent life. This presents the Manufacturing group with a range of potentially conflicting objectives which need to be managed within the overall product development context.

Increasing pressures on prices has led to pressure on margins and hence the need to understand the key costs in the process and ensure these are optimized. In this way profitability is maintained in the face of competition and price legislation.

Input from Manufacturing is now seen to start well before product launch right through to ultimate product withdrawal. Each phase of this life cycle presents different challenges to the project management structure.

More novel therapeutic approaches and presentations lead to more demands on Manufacturing and a need to understand every aspect of the process itself prior to launch to avoid technical problems and supply failure.

As overall corporate costs have come under pressure, the cost of infrastructure has been closely examined, and hence the number of facilities has been reduced. This places more demands on Development to ensure that the manufacturing process is robust and reproducible. Decisions about the location and type of plant in the light of the likely scale of the product are, therefore, critical.

All of these factors have combined to increase the demands made on Manufacturing and Manufacturing management. The process of product development must now be viewed in a holistic sense and Manufacturing can no longer be seen as an "add on" at the end of the development process. It must now be an integral part of the way in which a successful product is developed and introduced. It is essential that the key drivers of cost, supply logistics and, in the later stages of the product's life, competitive advantage through manufacturing innovation are well understood at the time that fundamental product decisions are being made. For branded products this becomes even more critical as patent expiry approaches. Generic threat can be turned into opportunity if the primary manufacturer understands the product, the process, and opportunities better than anyone else in the market. If OTC launch is contemplated, cost is also an important factor because price to the consumer is much more critical than if the molecule is a prescription product.

The key issues facing Manufacturing as a result of recent changes relate to their influence on the process of development and the degree of their involvement. Both primary and secondary Manufacturing need to be involved in numerous stages of the development of a product. The question is how should that involvement be triggered and by whom? There is a need for a well defined management process covering technical and commercial issues. This must interlock with the central R & D project structure and reflect the need for manufacturing project management and technical support structures. The purely physical operation of production is only one aspect of the activity. With pharmaceutical products, there are high risks and high rewards, and the triggering of actions in R & D, Marketing, and Manufacturing must be carefully considered before initiation. The balancing of expenditure against time and the risk of drug development is a crucial central role that must take place in Manufacturing as in all other units involved in development. To ensure that strategic decisions on investment timing and critical actions are well controlled, a business function is needed in Manufacturing, working alongside the production areas, to initiate relevant discussions and actions.

II. MANUFACTURING PHILOSOPHY

To meet the demands now placed on it, Manufacturing must alter the traditional stance frequency adopted toward involvement in product development. In addition, R & D also has to offer the optimum opportunity to involve Manufacturing in the process so as to achieve the best overall results for the organization. In the recent past a good deal of mutual suspicion existed between R & D and Manufacturing over the development process because of conflicting corporate objectives. For example, take the need for R & D process scale-up work in the manufacturing plant. This is not generally included in output figures for Manufacturing, hence reduces overall efficiency, and has often led to restricted access to the plant. R & D looked on Manufacturing as a secondary issue during development and has not tried to optimize production of the product, dealing instead with essentially scientific/medical issues as a priority for the dossier. Although this is quite correct from a restricted view, it misses the opportunity for close collaboration and improvements to launch with a right first-time dossier and right first-time process. Increasingly it is recognized that the key target is not the dossier submission but the realization of the product's commercial potential. Marketing has also contributed to a somewhat confrontational atmosphere by demanding the greatest possible flexibility in terms of presentations and the lowest cost design, thus challenging both R & D and Manufacturing in terms of the development program. All of this has often led to a situation where each unit tries to achieve conflicting objectives without trying to find the win:win situation that optimizes the overall outcome. Handling this conflict must begin at the top of the organization with the setting of appropriate strategic aims and shared objectives across functional boundaries. It can be argued, therefore, that good project management begins at the top by reducing the conflict of objectives and helping to set the agenda for collaboration.

Manufacturing can take its place at the drug development negotiating table in such a collaborative environment. It is no longer possible to stand apart from the process of developing the product and merely react as the approval for sale is achieved. Involvement in the process of development must be as a partner in the decision-making process accepting that not all outcomes are optimal for Manufacturing but are optimal for the overall product development effort. This requires a new breed of Manufacturing management and staff. They must have an intimate knowledge of the development process so that they take part in every stage of decision making and have a positive attitude toward the opportunity that innovation brings to them in new processes. Having a good strategic sense of the needs of the market and working in partnership with Marketing is also essential. Manufacturing must now put in place the right structures to deal with the technical and commercial issues that arise during the development of the product. This means dealing with a wide range of objectives, which can be conflicting, and seeking to optimize the overall outcome rather than any part of the process.

III. MANY CONFLICTING OBJECTIVES

As a result of the changing demands described above and with Manufacturing playing a positive part in development, they will face many and often conflicting objectives. The key ones are the following:

to collaborate with R & D to develop a robust and reproducible process which will meet the worldwide demand for the product, regulatory authorities' demands for data, and cost constraint targets.

the potential to provide material to development before the process is fully established but at the same time ensure that the product, which is eventually registered, can be manufactured to specifications capable of consistent reproduction.

to introduce a flexible production configuration, producing many different, value added, product variants without excessively raising costs. This can often be best achieved through the additions to lines which increase flexibility and increase brand image, e.g., on line tablet printing.

the ability to progressively improve the process over time to meet the needs of different points in the life cycle of the product, especially in the face of increased competition.

to supply worldwide demand for the product from the minimum number of plants with optimum distribution cost and delivery time to the market. Therefore, managing of the supply chain itself is a consideration as the product is developed. This has many ramifications for plant size, location, and make or buy decisions.

This represents a wide combination of objectives which individually are very challenging and combined demand diverse skills from Manufacturing. On the one hand, technical excellence is needed to produce material of a suitable standard for development or sale and to ensure that the optimum process is developed. On the other hand, good commercial understanding is needed to address the logistical issues of supply and cost and the strategic decisions related to risk, time, and cost tradeoffs. Any system of project management established in Manufacturing must meet all of these needs and ensure that none are neglected during the process.

IV. THE CHANGING DEMANDS OF EACH PHASE OF PRODUCT DEVELOPMENT

Manufacturing involvement in product development and the life cycle of the product is the only one that never ends (see Table 1). Active development of a molecule by R & D and Marketing ceases when there is no incremental income to be made from the product. Even operating unit marketing groups may stop supporting/detailing a declining product. However, for as long as the product remains on the sales list and orders are received, Manufacturing must continue to support the process. Contracting out may be used to reduce the demands but even then internal technical support is needed. The life cycle of the product in Manufacturing, therefore, can be

TABLE 1

Manufacturing Involvement by Phase

Stage of development	Role of manufacturing group	Likely membership	Issues
Molecule selection	Maintain awareness, monitoring, evaluating implications	Central Manufacturing Project management group	New processes, formulations, long term plant and machinery, implications of new technology uses
Preclinical Phase I/II	Active involvement in primary process development Monitoring secondary issues	Central Project Management, primary development team	Least-cost process, make or buy decision, plant, location of production
Phase II/III	Further refinement of primary process, full secondary development	Central Project Management, primary and secondary development teams	Final stages of primary process, secondary pack and process development (Market entry) Planning
Phase IV/ launch	Commence introduction of formulation and pack variants; full support to the market	Central Project Management Secondary development team	New formulations introduced, new pack designs Improving capacity management
Full commercialization Patent expiry		Central Project Management	Process patents, monographed specs New innovative formulations and pack designs

very long and the various different phases of development and commercialization make different demands on the manufacturing project management system.

Prior to phase I the involvement of Manufacturing is likely to be an information-only basis. This means, however, that all projects must still be actively monitored. An effective system is needed to point out issues which arise and to ensure intimate contact with the details of the product development process. The opportunity to intervene in the debate must always be there and must be actively sought if issues arise that affect manufacturing in the future. For example, the sourcing of a key and yet scarce raw material is crucial even at a very early stage of development and requires purchasing expertise from the Manufacturing function.

The involvement of the Manufacturing group begins in earnest in the early stages of drug development (i.e., around phase I/II), especially if the program is large and a very aggressive time scale is being pursued. The quantities of material required may mean that a plant scale campaign is needed to satisfy the demand even at this very early stage. There is also need for early involvement to look at a number of primary process issues, for example,

> the least cost design of the process and the potential routes that can be used to improve robustness and reproducibility;
>
> environmental and waste management issues which affect the final process, especially where these have quite a profound effect on company costs. Large waste management plants represent a considerable capital investment, and eliminating the need can often only be done early in the development process. For example, elimination of certain solvent or catalyst residues is achieved through alternative routes.
>
> plant and machinery needs with very long lead times. Lead times up to two years are not unknown, especially in the biotech field, where approval of the configuration by regulatory authorities takes some time to achieve.

At this stage, involvement of the primary manufacturing team at a technical level is crucial, with lesser involvement for the commercial functions, i.e., Planning/Project Management. Even at this very early stage, however, the Manufacturing staff involved in the project must bear in mind the issues related to the supply of the product on a large scale and avoid compromising later decisions. Another key issue is one of timing relative to the eventual regulatory submission. Some process issues are critical even at the early stage of development. As Manufacturing becomes involved in the primary process issues, the route of manufacture has an intimate relationship with the eventual dossier. Clearly, if manufacture of material for chronic toxicology and carcinogenicity studies takes place by a certain route, this cannot be changed later in the program without further work and potential time delays. The carcinogenicity study start date is the key watershed, the route intended for market must be final by then, with a fixed and well-understood impurity pattern. This leads to a submission for a route that must be supported by primary production and the equipment available, minimizing the need for immediate change after approval. Involvement with Chemical Development in the production of material for six-month animal studies and beyond is obviously a crucial interaction in ensuring the shortest possible overall development time. There is some secondary manufacturing involvement, especially where a novel dosage form is envisaged, such as a new type of solid dosage form or an inhaler. Secondary Manufacturing, therefore, has to be informed about the development and take part in key decisions about its dosage form/pack design, but may not wish to become fully involved at this very early stage where it is highly possible that the molecule will fail.

As development progresses into late phase II and phase III, the involvement of Manufacturing inevitably grows and this is the point at which they must be fully represented on the project. The involvement of Primary Manufacturing remains, of course, and with the R & D team, they will have begun finalization of the process which will be used in the final dossier. Around phase III and leading up to the initial submission, a number of important issues must be dealt with, for example,

process scale up and tailoring this to the plant available with appropriate validation of the reproducibility;

make or buy decisions where technically it may be easier for a specialist contractor to take on a particular part of the process rather than investing in-house;

the relationship with the secondary process in terms of specifications for the drug substance, e.g., particle size or moisture content.

In addition to the above primary process technical issues, a wide range of commercial issues also arise now which relate to the drug substance, for example,

Where should manufacturing be located to optimize costs and simplify logistical considerations while supporting secondary production to an optimal degree? Can nursery production plants be used initially to help stabilize the process prior to transfer into main production sites?

What is the likely demand for the eventual product? How will this be serviced and does this raise significant purchasing issues?

Is plant investment needed to support the expected peak demand?

During this period of development, the secondary manufacturing process will be under full-scale investigation to establish

a reproducible process tailored to the likely scale of demand. This is obviously proportionately more complex where sterile or specialist manufacture is needed;

the pack requirements, the number of possible variants and the purchasing specification of the materials involved;

the supply chain logistics for products where, for example, shelf life or storage conditions may be critical;

the location of secondary manufacturing. Whereas in primary manufacturing the number of locations used may be relatively limited, the number of secondary factories may be quite numerous and a process must be defined which is qualified in each plant, even where the facilities are relatively less sophisticated than those in the company's principal plants.

The involvement of Secondary Manufacturing in these areas is now vital and has to deal with the technical and commercial issues related to worldwide supply. Once again there are issues during this phase that are time-critical for the overall submission. The choice of pack types, for example, and the setting up of the relevant stability studies to support the submission are critical. Although the number of options for most dosage forms is limited and relatively easily dealt with, new presentations or new materials may create more critical problems. A new inhaled product with a novel dosing arrangement may involve considerable pack development, engineering, and machine supplier support with long lead times. Hence, timing the involvement of Secondary Manufacturing, especially in a pack engineering sense, is crucial to ensure that what goes into the submission in pack specifications is supportable.

After the product launch, manufacturing issues continue to multiply to support the product roll-out worldwide. There are many factors to be considered relative to plant size and location. Plant capacity clearly has to relate to market size, which is often a moving target. In the initial phase of introduction, demand is relatively moderate and requires a small-scale production unit to service the demand. This requires setting up a nursery production unit to help initial market entry with the option of some expanded capacity as demand rises. In addition to providing market entry stock, such a facility is used extensively during formulation and process development to define and test the manufacturing method proposed. This provides stability test material and the extensive amounts of material required for phase

III's clinical studies. To be utilized successfully and cost effectively, a nursery production facility needs equipment ensuring that the reduced scale manufacture is representative and provides a home for "future technology" investigations. The plant management process should clearly recognize that pharmaceutical R & D development work is one of its major customers as well as providing commercial material. This further contributes to the collaboration at an early stage and reduces the need for last-minute process modifications as market entry batches are manufactured.

The launch phase may involve a number of new dosage forms to increase penetration into the available market. Even at this very early stage of the product's life cycle, cost reduction and process optimization should be going on. At all times during the product's life cycle, the primary inventor of the molecule seeks greater expertise than anybody else in producing the entity. Very demanding specifications may be used as a potential barrier to entry, especially where they are monographed. Hence the organization must continue to address the process innovatively to improve the value-creating potential of the product constantly. The leadership of this activity should be Manufacturing itself and hence the project management system required will change to take more of a leadership role in partnership with R & D and Marketing. There also needs to be a clear partnership between Regulatory and Manufacturing functions to ensure that the product is consistently manufactured in conformance with worldwide product registrations and changing regulatory needs.

In the mature and declining phases of a product's patent life, the involvement of Manufacturing is even more crucial if the revenue from major products is to be defended as much as possible against competitive and generic erosion. The patent expiry defense strategy should be in place long before the patent actually expires to create barriers to market entry. Although this has only limited success, retaining the revenue from a top-twenty–selling prescription product, even for a short period, is worth a great deal of money to the organization. Strategies for defending the revenue include

switching the molecule to the OTC market, where possible, and building on the brand strength and recommender support acquired during the prescription life;

supply agreements with generic companies to control the introduction of unbranded versions of the drug and yet continue to generate a revenue stream for the original inventor;

lowest possible cost processes to compete with generics;

new patented process improvements;
new dosage forms which might be patentable and give some degree of protection from generic erosion, especially where they confer an additional clinical benefit over and above the molecule itself.

Involvement of Manufacturing in this late stage of the product's life is absolutely crucial and must lead in driving forward product changes which improve cost or patent protection. All such changes, of course, have R & D implications for supporting data and regulatory approval. Hence close liaison must be maintained through the project team structure and appropriate support within Manufacturing.

V. AN INTERLOCKING PROJECT STRUCTURE

Development programs and product introductions involve two groups of issues commercially related to cost, logistics, and supply, etc. and issues related to the technical development of the product itself. Both are, of course, linked and yet require different processes and different project management skills to deal with them adequately. In terms of interfaces, the commercial issues are very much linked to central and local Marketing regarding pack type, pricing, cost of goods, and demand for the product. The technical issues very much relate to the way in which R & D is developing the product, what is to be included in the dossier, and the support needed from R & D to improve the process after initial introduction. There are, of course, many issues where both coincide. For example, a decision by Marketing about the dosage form has a direct bearing on the R & D development program, which, in turn, has a major bearing on the way in which Manufacturing has to handle the product. Therefore, any approach to project management has to ensure that each issue is handled on its merits but also deals with areas of overlap.

Project Management is a relatively young discipline in the pharmaceutical industry, but increasingly the techniques are used to manage development projects. Part-time Project Leaders are also used in many companies, in conjunction with Project Managers or with strong planning support. In general there will always be a central project group with responsibility for planning and managing the development of a particular molecule and to whom the manufacturing aspects of the project must link seamlessly. To do this there must be a number of groups set up in Manufacturing responsible for integrating manufacturing into the overall project development.

The right representation of Manufacturing on the central project team is essential. These teams, most often led by R & D, are at one and the same time strategic and yet have to resolve a multitude of technical issues. However, the members of the team "represent" each function and are not generally expected to know every technical detail of their particular department's role. If one takes, as an example, the Clinical representatives, behind them are a number of other disciplines, e.g., statistics, data handling, whom they are expected to represent at team meetings (see Fig. 1).

To be effective, project group members need the following attributes:

broad understanding of the drug development process;
good appreciation of the role of their function in the development program and the role of the supporting functions in their area;
a broad understanding of the product and the technical issues likely to arise during the course of the project;
good communication and networking skills;

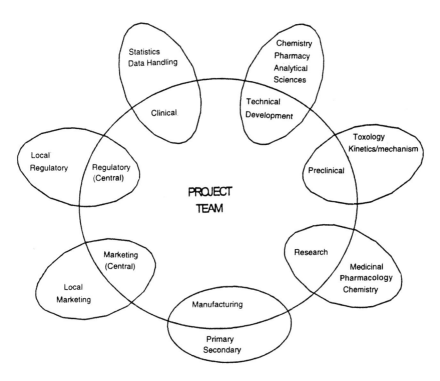

FIG. 1 Core product development team and supporting functions.

good understanding of the portfolio context of the project, the key objectives, and the target product profile.

Manufacturing is no exception to the above. Their representatives need these attributes to represent Manufacturing on the central project team and link with the R & D Project Leader and/or Project Manager. The Manufacturing project member must ensure that input into the overall project plan is given by the Manufacturing team and that, where timescales are critical, that these have been checked with the technical support teams to ensure feasibility. Quantities and demands on the process must also be established through liaison with central Marketing and also by the direct communication that Manufacturing often has the local marketing.

VI. MANUFACTURING PROJECT MANAGEMENT GROUP

Who should represent Manufacturing on the central project team? This question is often contentious within Manufacturing itself. On the one hand, the commercial areas (Planning/Purchasing, etc.) do not feel this should be left to the technical staff, and on the other hand, the technical staff does not feel that the commercial staff sufficiently understands the technical issues. Because the project team essentially ensures "representation" of all areas in the development process, this argues that technical specialism is not needed provided there is a strong technical support structure which has adequate links to the central R & D team. This in turn argues that the representative of Manufacturing on the team should be a skilled "Project Manager" rather than a technical expert.

At all stages of the development program and throughout the life cycle of the product, a good strategic view must be maintained on all aspects of the development of the manufacturing process, both technical and commercial. To do this, a group is needed that has essentially a commercial role in the organization which will organize the "business of manufacturing" but also ensure good links to physical production itself with the relevant technical support. This is the central Manufacturing Project Management Group.

This unit should be staffed by individuals with a broad understanding of all of the R & D, Development and commercial processes involved in bringing a product to the market. They also must be familiar with the company and the way in which both the formal and informal systems work, as it is their coordinating role that is most crucial in ensuring successful transfer of a product to production. Because it is quite rare to find individuals with the required skills in large numbers anywhere in the organization, a varied background group with skills drawn from R & D, Manufacturing and Marketing is the ideal approach. In this way the group has a collective strength of experience in many different areas of product development which make up for any individual lack of experience in any one area.

What role should the staff of this group play in the introduction of a product? First they must act as the member for Manufacturing on the central project team and ensure that they represent the interests of both the commercial and the technical staff. To do this they must possess the skills outlined above for the project group member and the leadership skills needed within the Manufacturing environment. One of the most crucial roles they must play is to appraise, on an ongoing basis, the timing of the project versus the cost of investment in Manufacturing, taking into account the relative risk at the phase of development. There are many tradeoffs in the timescale achievable, if risks are accepted through parallel rather than sequential processing to reduce timescale significantly. The Project Manager in Manufacturing needs to review constantly the relative risks of the project and the proposed investment in plant, machinery, raw materials, and intermediates. Recommendations must be made to both senior R & D and Manufacturing management, which balance the risks and costs, though this may affect timescales. An investment of many million in a relatively high-risk, moderate-reward project may not be advisable, whereas increased investment in a high-reward project may bring about significant improvements and lead to dramatically higher market rewards. With an "umbrella" view the Project Manager should be ideally positioned to make balanced recommendations based on advice from team members.

One area where this is of key importance is outsourcing. There is much more willingness now to consider this as an option than there has been in the past. Once upon a time, in-house production was likely to be preferred in most cases because of the perceived need to make full use of the facilities available in-company. However, now this philosophy has changed to take advantage of the wide range of specialized manufacturers now available. An example in the primary area is the use of specialists in chiral compound synthesis to avoid the need of investing in expensive process research and high plant costs (and indeed high risk). Outsourcing must be considered where the cost of processing is not justified by the potential return on investment. These are business decisions which require a thorough investment appraisal carried out on behalf of senior management, with appropriate recommendations on options to be considered. The Manufacturing Project Management Group is ideally placed to make these recommendations. This places further demands on the key skills required by this group to include contract negotiation and management, to ensure that optimal use is made of both in-house and contractor resources.

The Project Managers assigned to each project by Manufacturing has to ensure that they are acting in the right "context" and hence they must ensure that the basic parameters within which the project operates are clearly understood. To do this during the development phase, they must define for the Manufacturing staff a number of constraints, for example,

the target introduction date and the key milestones in the R & D program. This allows the Manufacturing groups to define their own key milestones for the production process, which are in line with the R & D program;

the portfolio priority of the project and hence the extent of resources that it should be given versus other projects if clashes arise;

total likely demand for the product, clearly established with Marketing, to ensure that both the primary and secondary processes are designed to meet the capacity required;

any constraints that there may be on the project, e.g., costs or specification limits.

After launch, the information needed by each group changes significantly and involves a definition of the long-term plan for the product, including:

demand over time,

country launch plans, and

launch dates for new formulations.

The Project Manager frequently acts as project "chair" for the technical transfer groups, though not necessarily for all of the project discussions, as it may be appropriate for someone from the technical team to do this on given technical issues. What the Project Manager must ensure is that all groups dealing with the same compound are adequately informed about progress to date and the proposed way in which cross-group issues are to be dealt with. The Project Manager is likely also to organize project reporting on progress to senior management and ensure that issues are highlighted for decisions that cannot be resolved at a project team level.

VII. THE TECHNICAL SUPPORT STRUCTURE

With a central Project Management team staffed by generalists who are essentially employed to look after the commercial/logistical aspects of the project and communication/coordination, a good technical support structure is also needed to ensure that the process is designed with manufacturing capabilities and any technical constraints in mind.

Two product transfer groups are needed to deal with the actual technical development of the process and its transfer into the primary and secondary manufacturing unit (see Fig. 2). Although they deal with different parts of the process it is important that they communicate well between them. Hence some common membership is advantageous, as well as some joint meetings where issues of interfaces between the teams are handled. The central Project Manager is a member of both teams and indeed probably acts as chairman of both for the main meetings.

The primary process handover team has two main objectives which cover numerous subissues:

to produce a safe, reproducible process which can be transferred to a number of plants around the world at a suitable cost of goods; the safety issue is crucial because, with increasing environmental protection legislation around the world, this issue has to be dealt with during the development process; and

to ensure that the dossier reflects the needs of primary manufacturing in terms of achievable specifications.

To achieve this, representation is needed from the Chemical and Analytical Development in R & D, primary plant management in Manufacturing, QA, Engineering, Environmental/Safety management and Purchasing. The central manufacturing Project Manager acts as the coordinator for the group to ensure that it understands the demands on the process, the priority of the project, and the overall plan being pursued by the R & D project team.

The secondary group is somewhat larger because it has to deal with many more issues and may indeed need to split into different subgroups if different dosage forms are needed. However, a core team is needed to coordinate all the detail of the program to ensure that it remains integrated across the full development. The composition of the secondary group obviously varies somewhat depending on the formulation, but comprises Secondary Manufacturing (e.g., tableting, sterile products), Packaging (the relevant packing unit), Pack design/engineering, Purchasing, Engineering and QA. Once again the Project Manager acts as the chair/coordinator of the group.

When should each group be formed? It is important that the structure and membership is in place as early as possible in the product's life cycle,

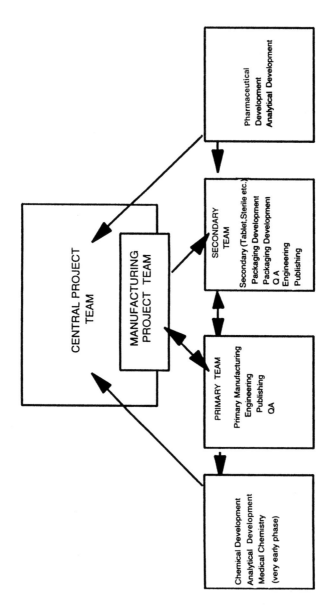

FIG. 2 Technical support structure.

even if the groups are not activated until a later date. The Project Manager, who is monitoring the project, must activate the groups at an appropriate time to ensure that adequate input is given on key manufacturing issues. In the meantime, the Project Manager must ensure a good flow of information to each group so it is fully prepared for the time when Manufacturing is fully involved.

Although the makeup of the groups is vital to high-quality input into the product development process and improving the flow of information within Manufacturing, the right process also needs to be put in place. Hence attention must be paid to the right level of objective setting, reporting on progress, and planning support. Clearly the project objective, personified in the target product profile, must reflect key manufacturing issues, especially where they set the parameters for the process. An example of this would be where a novel dosage form is needed to give a compound a competitive edge. Reporting must be done regularly to ensure that all key personnel in Manufacturing are informed of progress, not only at a senior management level, but also at an operational level where it is obvious that not everyone involved with a project can sit directly on the project team. Simple format reporting must be designed which minimizes bureaucracy and optimizes information.

Finally in planning, there are two basic options, decentralization and centralization. Decentralizing planning to set up a Manufacturing project planning system has some advantages of the plan being "owned" by Manufacturing itself. It also probably allows more detail to be put into the plan. However, in one sense this begins to reemphasize the separate nature of Manufacturing from the rest of the process. Centralizing planning has some advantages in that the key manufacturing milestones become an integral part of the overall development plan. Then it is still possible to do more detailed local planning to supplement the overall development plan. Using this approach also encourages central R & D planning to become more involved with the Manufacturing issues and hence help to support the Manufacturing Project Manager.

VIII. WORLDWIDE PRODUCTION

As with all Functions in the modern pharmaceutical company, Manufacturing is a worldwide activity. Companies usually have a number of primary manufacturing units and certainly numerous secondary manufacturing units. Decisions about where to locate production are likely to be based upon slightly differing considerations for the drug substance and the secondary pack. For the drug substance, the decision is as much financial as anything else. Tax breaks, low-cost manufacturing areas, etc. all play a part in determining the most appropriate location for the primary manufacturing site. For secondary production, the decision is slightly more complex and certainly involves a good deal of consideration of logistical, technical, and financial issues (especially transfer pricing and retained local profits). Tablet manufacturing and sterile production are concentrated in a few areas because of the technical issues that they raise and the high cost of such facilities. Packaging is much easier to transfer to a local market where some financial incentives are offered for locating at least part of the manufacturing in a given country.

Given the worldwide nature of manufacturing, it is important that a structure similar to the one described above is installed in all countries where products are to be introduced. The central Project Management team still acts in a strategic role to keep a tight control on the timing of introduction, but local teams are needed to ensure a smooth transfer into the local facility. The central product transfer group members assist in this process by ensuring that local staff is aware of particular technical issues that arose during development.

IX. SUMMARY

With increasing the complexity of the drug development process and with pressure on time and cost, a more holistic approach is needed to involve all functions and ensure that outcomes are optimized. Manufacturing must take a central role, along with R&D and Marketing, within the whole product development process. To do this, it must structure itself to optimize both technical and commercial input into crucial development decisions. Using a Project Management Group approach to act as a central coordinating body within Manufacturing, therefore, is recommended to ensure that technical involvement is orchestrated at the right time and business-related decisions are taken in the light of cost, risk, and time factors.

REFERENCES

T Hill, The Strategy Management of the Manufacturing Function, *Manufacturing Strategy*. Macmillan Press Ltd, 1992, pxy.

S Wheelwright, K Clark. Quantum Leaps in Speed, Efficiency and Quality, *Revolutionising Product Development*. Free Press, 1992, PXY.

11

Implementation of Project Management: Management of Change

Astrid H. Seeberg

The Bracco Group
Milan, Italy

I. INTRODUCTION

In this chapter we intend to illustrate a successful change in management using the case of Bracco Corporate. Bracco is a middle-sized pharmaceutical company, essentially family managed, and a leader in one area—contrast media for radiology. It is one of the very few, truly global, niche companies.

Bracco is a good example because the change it had to face was drastic and because its volume and overall focus in R&D make a detailed analysis feasible with reasonable effort.

Up to the late eighties, Bracco was an Italian-based research and manufacturing company, whose wealth came mainly from one blockbuster product, Iopamidol, created and manufactured by Bracco and sold worldwide through licensees (the compound still holds a leading position in the world market for nonionic X-ray contrast media).

Based on the success of Iopamidol and its accumulated excellence in R&D, manufacturing, and management, Bracco was ready for more; its aim is to become the world leader in contrast media for in vivo diagnosis by the year 2000 despite fierce competition and market turbulence.

II. WHY CHANGE?

To achieve such an ambitious target required that Bracco meet a number of challenges:

extending R&D into all areas of in vivo diagnostics (X-ray, magnetic resonance imaging (MRI) and ultrasound)

passing from sequential development to parallel development of several projects

starting portfolio management systems to select and prioritize the different projects

qualifying the Milan site as a true corporate head office of a global corporation

gaining direct marketing presence in all major markets

creating an international marketing organization to guide subsidiaries and distributors world-wide.

These challenges were met by

acquiring know-how and capacity in discovery, development, and manufacturing by purchasing and building sites in the U.S., Germany, and Switzerland

purchasing sales organizations and creating joint ventures in Europe (Bracco–Byk Gulden) and in Japan (Bracco–Eisai).

changing the management structure.

By the early nineties, Bracco had entered a true transitional period, changing from a national to an international, from a monoproduct to a product portfolio and from a single site to a globally present corporation.

III. CHANGE STARTS IN R&D

R&D has always been the fundamental business driver of the Group with heavy investment continuing and even increased. The corporation has given R&D a strong mission: to generate a wide range of innovative, high-value-added products in all areas of in vivo imaging with new product launches at least every two years in all major markets.

To meet these objectives, Bracco's management realized that a fundamental reorganization of the R&D structure and culture was indispensable in the medium term. The first target for reorganization was development. The objectives of the change in development were

to speed up development times through better organization and decision processes

to balance national requirements more efficiently against global development and product standardization

to better integrate changes in markets, medical needs, instruments and pharmaeconomics into the development process

to plan and control resources on a corporate level

to allow prioritization of projects and their timely termination.

The question of how best to organize corporate Discovery activities could be asked only after the process of acquiring discovery groups had been consolidated. This was in 1995 when the Bracco Group found itself with three research centers (Switzerland, Italy, and the U.S.), each managed independently with different approaches to Discovery. At this point an inventory of research activities and resources worldwide was generated. The result revealed that, although Bracco probably had the best contrast media researchers worldwide, the output of innovative molecules was low. The ratio of the total cost of Discovery to the total cost of R&D was too high. The targets for change in Discovery were identified as

a new changed process of Discovery

the avoidance of duplication of Discovery programs

the development of better processes for identifying "lead" development candidates

a method of accounting for all resources in well-defined programs.

IV. STEPWISE APPROACH TO INTRODUCING CHANGE INTO THE DEVELOPMENT ORGANIZATION

To assist the reader in better understanding the need for a prudent introduction of change, we have to come back to the background of Bracco.

Toward the end of the eighties and beginning of the nineties, Iopamidol sales peaked in all major markets. The company grew enthusiastically and the atmosphere inspired a great sense of pride and security. In this period, however, Bracco's traditional competitor Schering launched its first contrast medium in a new imaging modality, magnetic resonance imaging, and voices were also being heard about Nycomed being launched shortly.

It was then that the first doubts about Bracco's competitiveness arose, especially with regard to the time required to develop a new contrast medium. Project Management was proposed as a managerial tool to gain time. Soon afterwards, in 1991, an outsider with experience in preclinical and clinical development was employed in the position of Pilot Project Leader. The first move toward a matrix organization had been made (see Table 1 for a summary of the changes).

TABLE 1
Changes in R&D, Bracco Group

1991 Weak Matrix Local Development Trial: first Project	Step 1: One Pilot Project Leader Milan
↓ *Europeization*	
1992 Weak Matrix EU Development	Step 2: Seven development projects, Milan, Geneva, coordination Japan, Executive Committee R&D, Director Project Planning and Head of Project Coordination
↓ Trial: Multiproject	
1995 Weak Matrix Worldwide	Step 3: Nine development projects, each with a Team in the U.S. and Europe and an Executive Committee R&D with U.S. and European delegates; Development Director with international budget responsibility; Heads of Project Management in EU and U.S.
↓ Trial: Worldwide projects *Globalization*	
↓ *Extension to research and centralization*	
1996 Strong Matrix in R&D	Step 4: Nine international development projects guided by central International Project Leader with full responsibility for time and resources Research organized in programs with Program Leader R&D led by Co-Director "Portfolio" and Co-Director "Resources" Corporate Project Planning, Strategic Product Group at headquarters

Step 1: Weak matrix in local development and nomination of
        Pilot Project Leader

The main purpose of this figure was to bring the activities of one highly promising project together. A planning software Winproject, selected because of its ease of use, was introduced. The Project Leader coordinated personally to get the rather hierarchically rooted line managers used to the "change."

A team was established and investment made in teamwork training. The team suffered from a lack of delegation by line managers and a lack of decision making power. Nevertheless, valuable experience was collected in this period.

Step 2: Project Management in Europe,
        start multiproject management

Bracco continued to grow, extending beyond the Italian border. The company acquired a research group in Geneva, Switzerland (now Bracco Research Geneva) and formed joint ventures in Germany (Bracco–Byk Gulden) and Japan (Bracco–Eisai). The research groups in Switzerland and Italy flourished, proposing several molecules (six) for development. At this point it became obvious that Development needed to be reorganized to handle activities at several sites and manage a number of projects in parallel.

The President, therefore, established a new function dedicated entirely to Project Planning and Management. The following matrix structures were created:

Executive Committee (CERS)

Composition: Directors of Research sites (Milan, Geneva), Director Project Planning and Development, Medical Director Milan. Chairman Director R&D.

Tasks: Selection of development candidates with indications, company time targets and territories, major milestone decisions, project strategy and priority after consultation with local marketing functions; periodic project review, endorsement of Project Leaders.

Head of Project R&D Co-ordination

Responsible for structure, training and multiproject management.

Project Leader

Tasks: Coordination of project activities; responsibility for the realization of the project's aims and represents the project within the Bracco Group.

Project Planning: Activities, milestones, decision points, time lines, risks in accordance with project strategy and priority; commitment and resources from line managers.

Project Performance: time tracking, identify issues and chase problems, ensure continuous commitment by line managers, ensure team dynamic per phase, invite temporary members, organize external presentations, prepare project dossier, minutes, keep collection of major documents (protocols, reports, presentations).

In all, seven Project Leaders were installed. They remained in the line function and were expected to dedicate about 30 percent of their time to managing the project. The Head of R&D Coordination organized training sessions and supported the Project Leaders in their activities. This function also facilitated transferring project experience from one project to another and enabled monitoring general performance.

The scope of Project Management and the roles of the Project Leaders were defined in a Project Manual.

Experience:

The reporting structure and decision process on projects improved considerably.

Realistic (almost) time plans were achieved

Teams functioned best when:

international (the power of individual local Line Managers was less) empowered managers were delegated as Team Members

Project Leaders were senior staff with superior technical knowledge of the project and a clear vision of its potential.

Although the Project Management structure was received as a shock in 1992, by mid 1995 it was an everyday reality because of the patience and personal skills of the Project Leaders.

Step 3: Project Management Worldwide

1995

After the acquisition of Squibb Diagnostics from Bristol Meyers Squibb (now Bracco Diagnostics (BDI) and Bracco Research USA) a new international structure was required which took account of the diversity of experience at the EU and the U.S. development sites. Whereas Bracco Milan had been strongly R&D oriented but with no sense of urgency, BDI Project Management was strongly business-linked with a tendency to favor time over scientific depth. The BDI Project Leaders were employees of the Market Development Department and worked full time on Project Management, whereas the European Project Leaders were on loan from line functions.

In establishing a consistent worldwide structure, we took the best from both continents and installed a dual Project Management system with each Project Team managed by two distinct figures: an International Project Leader and a Project Manager.

Each team is now led by an international, highly visionary Project Leader whose responsibility is to develop the compound to its fullest potential worldwide. The International Project Leader is responsible for generating a Strategic Development Plan and the share-out of activities worldwide. He/she remains in his/her position as senior Line Manager. The International Project Leader is supported by a Process Manager who manages the day-to-day project work and the "chasing up." There is one International Team Leader worldwide and a Local Team Leader per project plus process managers in the EU and the U.S. local teams.

Major insights were obtained during this period:

Only very experienced highly visionary and senior managers (European level of seniority: Director or U.S.: Vice President) are capable of leading worldwide projects.

Project Managers are necessary to reduce the workload of the Project Leader and to ensure the "follow up" on the decisions of the team

Centralized strategic marketing input is necessary for the global vision; local marketing input is not sufficient.

Resources need to be managed project by project.

Priorities have to be set centrally.

V. STRUCTURE OF R&D AFTER CHANGE (1996)

After five years of trials, the corporation was convinced that the matrix system was *the* system to ensure Bracco's future. R&D was fully confirmed as the corporate "business" driver. The major features are summarized in Fig. 1.

All worldwide Discovery and Development activities are covered by a matrix comprising a Pipeline organization (with Co-Director "Pipeline") and a resource organization (Co-Director Resources).

The Pipeline organization is responsible for R&D output. All Project Leaders (PL for Development) and Program Managers (PM for Discovery) report directly to the Pipeline Director. The key features which determine the Pipeline organization include the right of the PL/PM to acquire resources

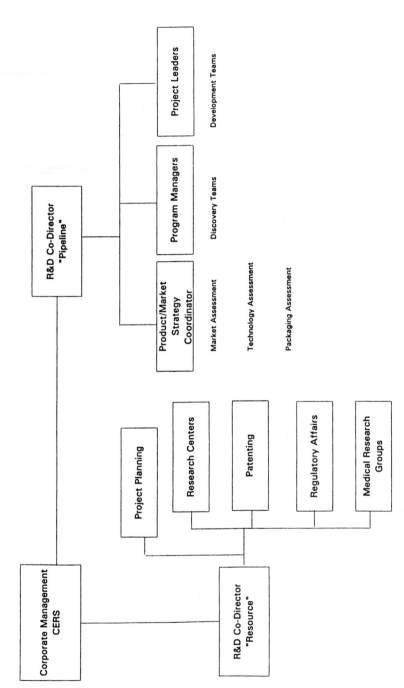

FIG. 1 Organization of R&D. CERS: Executive Committee Research and Development.

from the most appropriate competence centers worldwide, to evaluate team composition during the life cycle of the project, and to evaluate Team Members' performance. Strategic compliance is ensured by the worldwide Product/Market Strategy Group which reports to the Pipeline Director. Strategic decisions are made by the CERS and General Management.

The Pipeline Director has the mission of ensuring that a sufficient number of the "right" products get to the market before competitors and that the Discovery and Development Pipeline are adequately fed.

The Pipeline organization finds its Matrix partner in the Resource organization. The Resource Director has authority and responsibility for ensuring the availability of the resources needed (people, infrastructures, systems, third parties) for R&D output and for designing, integrating, and controlling the related development plan and budget.

Competencies are organized as areas of technological and process specialization:

Competence Centers, organized for example as Chemistry, Biochemistry departments. Every R&D person belongs to a Competence Center.

Project Planning ensures the allocation of adequate competencies to projects based on their priority and provides overall multiproject resource scheduling support.

The key figures of the new organization are described below.

Project Leader

Role: executes the assigned project on time, within budget and to the right standards of Quality, managing all required activities, resources, and budget. The Project Leader is a very senior employee with a major line responsibility (Director of Research Center, Medical Affairs, or a Competency Area).

Responsibilities of the Project Leader:

Is in charge of all Development activities for the assigned project
Puts together the Core Team and International Subteams and defines the Project Work Plan
Manages the program budget and progress.

Program Manager

Role: responsible for the scientific content of the research programs and their outcomes. He/she has very strong technical know-how in a program area.

Responsibilities: The PM defines program work plans in accordance with the Discovery Plan. He/she

manages the program budget and progress and assigned program resources
guarantees the correct analysis of the patent situation
promotes the positive image of Bracco in the scientific community
is responsible for preparing and sponsoring the business case.

All Bracco R&D employees are now organized in a Project or Program with complete accountability and transparency of resources. The thinking process in Discovery is changing from one directed towards fulfilling a task to one of reaching a milestone.

VI. PHILOSOPHY OF THE CHANGE PROCESS

Bracco is a traditional company. Business decisions (and all other decisions) are usually made after a period of maturation. They are based on in-depth analysis and experience and are rarely influenced by managerial fashions. This culture is also reflected in the stepwise introduction of changes in R&D management.

The nomination of the first Project Leader was a true trial run and, if it had been unsuccessful, could easily have been undone. Its success, however, encouraged expanding the Project Leader concept to incorporate seven project team leaders and the nomination of a dedicated Director, etc.

Seven development projects were closely observed by management and their strengths and shortcomings analyzed. This resulted in the Group "leaping" to Step 4.

Steps 1–3 can be described as a forced evolution, forced by the immense growth and internationalization of Bracco. These changes were, at least to some extent, reactive.

Step 4, however, is proactive, directed to the future. In fact, the fundamental reengineering of all R&D functions is a small revolution. Comforted by the positive experience in the previous evolution, the Bracco corporation had committed itself to a new R&D approach.

12

Information Technology and Future Visions of Pharmaceutical Project Management

Ian Trout, Paul H. Willer, Andrew J. M. Black, Helen Grant, and Nick Edwards

Andersen Consulting
Manchester and London, England

Additional contributions from: Pradip Banerjee, Jan Paul Zonnenberg, Mary Jo Veverka, Gale Thompson, George Smith, Kay Renfrew, Patrick Howard, Anatole Gershman, David Hadley, Stephen Sato, Kishore Swaminathan, and Mark Edwards.

I. INTRODUCTION

The pharmaceuticals industry is facing an increasingly competitive future. The ever mounting internal and external pressures on the industry are forcing companies to seek new and revolutionary ways of doing business. "Business as usual" is not an option.

The drug development process is no exception as the quality and quantity of the R&D pipelines come under greater scrutiny. To successfully respond to these pressures, the heads of pharmaceutical R&D organizations need to utilize their people and associated supporting technology more effectively. Alongside this, information technology (IT) continues to develop at an astounding rate enabling many new and innovative ways of working.

As the volumes of information required within a drug development project grow, the need to better develop, collate and manage it has never been more important. To handle much of this information, IT is being successfully deployed but, generally, in a localized departmental or functional fashion. A more integrated use of IT across geographical and departmental boundaries is needed to provide better handling and management of the information through the entire process. This would provide information for project management to enable appropriately informed decisions in a timely manner.

This chapter addresses how IT is used today in managing a drug development project and introduces the major technological developments which are starting to impact this area. In view of these developments, the future of drug development projects and their management is explored.

II. TODAY'S USE OF INFORMATION TECHNOLOGY IN DRUG DEVELOPMENT

Information technology has fast become a crucial factor in the success of the drug development process. As a result, significant investment is now committed to its support and development. However, these IT systems have not been developed as an integrated whole.

IT existing within drug development can be broken down into three broad categories:

- Personal productivity tools. This includes tools, such as word processors, graphics packages, spreadsheets, etc. that are used as standalone applications on the desktop to assist individuals in their day to day tasks.

- Localized departmental systems. Localized IT systems have been built by departments/functions to support their processes and tasks. In many cases, this has been done in an isolated manner, with the interfaces to the other areas of the drug development process receiving secondary consideration. In these scenarios, rather than facilitating integration, IT is a barrier between departments and to the flow of the overall process.
- Communications facilities. This includes tools which support communication between individuals. Currently, electronic mail provides the main communication channel but this is mainly used for ad hoc, unstructured communication. With a strong lead from management, electronic mail has revolutionized working environments enabling circulation of news, information and copies of documents to many recipients at the touch of a button. Unfortunately, the ease and speed of spreading information via electronic mail is easily abused. Information saturation is fast becoming commonplace, and, as a result, valuable information is being lost.

Figure 1 illustrates the typical fragmented set of IT tools with which members of a drug development project are faced. Typical team members (User) have access to stand-alone personal productivity tools local to the PC. They also have access to one or more departmental systems. This enables them to work with certain information in conjunction with other team members inside the department (and relies heavily on colocation) but is of little use outside it. Finally, the typical user also has access to some kind of communication capability, typically electronic mail. This facilitates interdepartmental, intersite and even intercompany communication.

IT solutions are reinforcing functional and geographical boundaries and the lack of use by senior management emphasizes any bureaucracy. Thus islands of information develop, as illustrated in Fig. 2.

In an attempt to break down these barriers, groupware is emerging to build additional capabilities around electronic mail and link personal productivity tools to support collaboration and information sharing between individuals, e.g., workflow, discussion forums, etc. This can provide a more structured way to share information than electronic mail. At the moment within the pharmaceuticals arena, groupware has been implemented, primarily, as a departmental system and has not been widely deployed across geographical boundaries.

Fortunately, some progress is being made to provide IT support for information sharing during the drug development process. Document man-

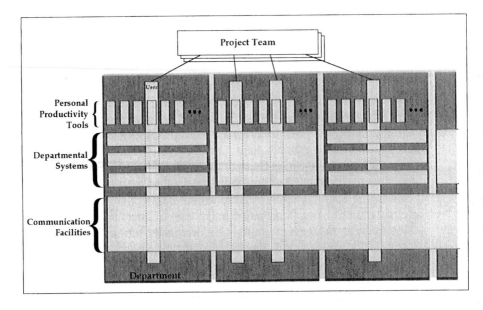

FIG. 1 IT today in a typical pharmaceutical company.

agement is a key enabler to providing a structured environment for information sharing. Concurrent development—where multiple parties work on different aspects of the same deliverables during the same time period—is possible because the system controls who has access to what and

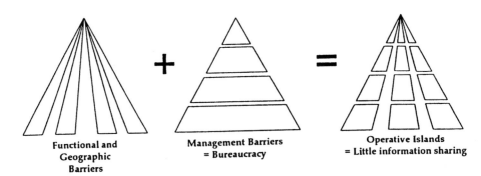

FIG. 2 Islands of information.

when. This ensures that data integrity and version control are properly maintained.

In the late 1980s, the FDA initiative to promote Computer Aided New Drug Applications (CANDAs), suggested strong movement towards integrated systems with a final electronic deliverable. For a variety of reasons, progress has not been as fast as originally hoped. Today, the compilation and submission of clinical trial data alone is often termed a CANDA. Without integrated systems, compiling an electronic submission can be as manually intensive as the paper process.

Beyond these developments in document management and groupware, use of integrated systems has been limited, particularly within project management. Project management in drug development has been treated, primarily, as a separate administrative function with little autonomy or authority over financial, personnel or time-line issues. This function is generally focused on dealing with project planning and tracking. The IT which supports it is another example of a stand-alone system. In reality, it is little more than an additional personal productivity tool on the desktop, sitting next to the word processor or graphics package. In some organizations where the requirement for more integrated project management has been identified, more sophisticated and specialized (and significantly more expensive) packages have been used to provide vertical integration. These packages provide "roll-up" capabilities to integrate different project plans. This gives an overall picture of the organization's drug development pipeline. Unfortunately, these systems are not renowned for their user-friendliness or level of functionality compared with the more generic, mass-market, stand-alone project management tools. The more sophisticated systems often provide project tracking information for senior management but are of little use to the project manager. This often means that the project manager maintains information on two systems, leading to significant inaccuracies and data integrity issues.

Compounding this problem further, the exchange and collection of information is frequently carried out manually. Many organizations use isolated project management teams to collect and enter the data. The quality of information supplied to these teams is generally poor and the processes of data collection, input, and production can be lengthy. Consequently, the collated information is often out-of-date, inaccurate, and cannot be relied upon for critical management decisions, and this has a crucial impact on project management. Any inaccuracies are further compounded when roll-up is used to provide a broader R&D picture.

At a higher level, project management also requires effective management of the business case and allocation of resources:

- Business case management. Maintaining the balance between scientific and commercial viability has not been an easy concept for R&D departments. But it has become essential to recognize the increasing importance of managing the business case at key milestones throughout a development project to ensure that critical decisions are timely and that all implications are known as the key drivers change. It is no longer acceptable to create the business case at the beginning of the development cycle and, then, leave it to one side. There are IT tools today which can assist the "what if" analysis process of managing the business case. However, these are not widely employed.
- Resource management/capacity planning. Managing the allocation of people across projects has always been difficult and, with the growing pressure to reduce head counts, it is important to improve this process. Some of the bigger project management IT tools mentioned earlier in the chapter provide resource management but suffer because the detailed data entered at the project level are inaccurate. At present, little use is made of IT to capture historical information and use it as a benchmark for future projects.

Supplying precise, current information to project management processes and monitoring key drivers are essential if critical decisions are to be made with any accuracy. This is imperative for the successful pharmaceutical companies of tomorrow which will have to work with much slimmer margins and tighter timescales.

Pharmaceutical companies have made a significant investment in IT and have reaped substantial benefits using it. No organization is fortunate enough to have a clean sheet on which to start. For the successful deployment of new technology, it is essential that appropriate consideration is given to integration with existing systems.

III. MAJOR IT DEVELOPMENTS

The constant evolution of IT is rapidly providing new opportunities for business solutions. As prices fall, these technologies also become increasingly viable for organizations to implement. The effect of IT on business operations can be traced through the past 30 years (see Fig. 3).

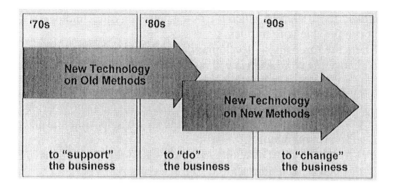

FIG. 3   The effect of IT on business operations.

Throughout the 1970s, IT, or data processing as it was called, was used primarily to automate business support functions, such as accounting. The 1980s saw the applications emerge to automate business functions themselves, for example, sales. IT remained focused on automating clerical, systematic processes that were routine and repeatable. Personnel employed within these areas have now embraced IT as a necessary part of their daily operations. Because of the nature of work involved in bringing a drug to market, IT did not have a major impact on the drug development processes at that time.

In the early 1990s, IT applications emerged which, for the first time, have had an impact on the knowledge worker. The term "knowledge worker" refers to a person who applies specialized business knowledge to business tasks, i.e., most of the people in the drug development process. These applications have primarily taken the form described in the previous section: personal productivity tools (including the project planning tools, word processors and spreadsheets used by the project manager) and communication capabilities.

At times, implementing these new applications has been a painful process because user requirements and expectations were mishandled. To a large extent, this has laid the groundwork for the future because knowledge workers are beginning to view IT as an intrinsic part of their daily lives (and not merely part of someone else's). The increasing spread of technology into people's homes has also played a positive role in promoting extensive daily use of IT at work. However, there are still big steps to be taken to gain full advantage of the support which the new generation of technological innovation can provide core business processes.

There are three major developments in IT which, together, are emerging to change the way business will operate:

- Integration. The ability to connect different systems to allow interaction and consolidation of the information used and provide support across the business process regardless of departmental and geographical boundaries.
- Virtual entities. The ability to create digital representations of people, places, and objects.
- Interactive Reach. The ability to reach people and organizations, interactively in real time.

This is illustrated in Fig. 4.

A. Integration

Integration is an essential first step in resolving many of the difficulties impeding the effective use of IT in the pharmaceutical industry today. This is happening for two major reasons. First, senior management increasingly

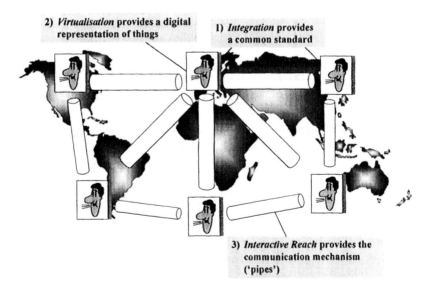

FIG. 4   The three major IT trends.

recognizes the significant value in standards and consistency across projects, functions, and at a global enterprisewide level. The implementation of standards enables easier exchange of information with or without IT. In parallel with this, the IT industry is moving to more "open" architectures and standards that allow communication of information between isolated systems. The proprietary systems of five to ten years ago have no place in today's corporate environment.

Integration will enable IT to provide solutions to support the drug development process in its entirety and assist in breaking down barriers between functions and other project teams. IT will facilitate the exchange of information enterprisewide, essential for success in tomorrow's global pharmaceutical industry. No pharmaceutical company today can afford to reinvent the wheel. The reuse of corporate knowledge is critical.

Integration will provide a logical repository of information stored in a consistent format and will allow transparent access across functional and geographical boundaries. Individuals can have a filtered, tailored view of the information appropriate to their tasks, thus, avoiding the problems of information saturation.

Furthermore, there is now an increased emphasis on using object-oriented technology to create modular systems. Each part of the system—for example, the user interface or the applications which actually perform business functions—is a separate "black box." A system is made of multiple modules linked together. Reuse is encouraged, change can be localized and controlled, and new interfaces and business functions can easily be incorporated into the system. Perhaps most important, object-oriented systems mirror the business functions of the organizations they serve. So they are easier to understand than traditional data processing systems.

B. Virtual Entities

The ability to create digital representations of people, places, and objects leads to an increase in the accuracy and flexibility of information stored and manipulated electronically. Digital representations of information allow these representations to be sent between locations and to exist in several locations simultaneously.

This technology has been used in a limited way for several years—consider the examples of flight simulation and on-line shopping. However, the technology can be applied in many other instances with few limitations (it has been estimated that three-quarters of processes/objects can be digitized), leading to dramatic changes in the way we use information at work and at home. For example, it will be possible to collect, analyze, and present information continuously, to tailor available information to personal, specific needs, and to have superior yet cheaper access to products, services, people, and capital.

C. Interactive Reach

The ability to reach people and organizations interactively in real time, together with virtualization, is eliminating the physical constraints of space, time, and form. This means that team members can share distributed information and resources, participate in distributed processes, and interact as if they were working next to each other. In effect, a workplace can be virtually created for each worker wherever located. This will have a profound impact on the way we conduct our business and social lives.

On a personal level, the reduced travel brought about by this application of technology will provide a more stable lifestyle for employees. At the same time, the ability to "talk" to colleagues on the other side of the world, as-needed, will promote the sense of belonging to one global firm.

Direct benefits include cheaper offshore development, reduced travel expenses, and a reduction in productive time lost on planes and suffering from jet lag. Indirect benefits may include less rework (as people will find it much easier to find out what other colleagues in the company have done before) and greater quality of work (the ability to "stand on the shoulders of giants" by building on global test practices). The net result will lead to reduced development time and increased consistency and quality of product.

Implementing and applying these technologies will provide many challenges. Organizations need to ensure they recognize the human factors which may be lost if IT is implemented without thought for people and process. To fully integrate IT into the business requires establishing a clear strategy with consideration of people, processes, and technology (see Fig. 5).

The convergence of computing, communications, and knowledge is already being used powerfully. For example, the Internet demonstrates all three technological trends and is expanding astronomically, providing a wealth of opportunities in the commercial sector and to private users.

Internet solutions have always been made up of individual technology services and standards that interoperate efficiently and effectively. The Internet is clearly focused on the "outside world" and is the quintessential end-user driven technology. The corporate Internet, the Intranet, is being used within organizations as another mechanism for collaboration and in-

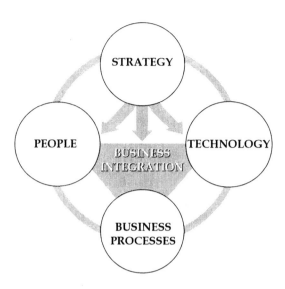

FIG. 5 The business integration model.

formation sharing. Intranet technology is a fast growing area, starting to be used by many of the world's largest companies, which have discovered that Web technology can improve information sharing across their networks.

In summary, these technologies will lead to greater access and control of information, a valuable resource in the pharmaceutical industry today.

IV. FUTURE VISIONS OF DRUG DEVELOPMENT

There is significant potential for leveraging IT to obtain substantive changes in the pharmaceutical industry. But to focus on the implementation of IT as a sole enabler would be misplaced. There is no doubt that new developments in IT will provide significant opportunities, but simultaneous consideration of people and process is also necessary to achieve the desired business goals. Too often, companies disregard the fact that their business processes may need to change, and their people may struggle to accept any changes without appropriate consultation.

Fortunately, in line with the IT developments, new ways of working are impacting the way projects will be managed. The major new approaches are

- cross-functional high-performance teams.

- globalization
- virtual organizations.

A. Cross-Functional High-Performance Teams

Over a number of years, there has been a drive towards new organizational forms. The realization that better results are achieved by skilled, motivated, focused teams has resulted in a growing trend toward empowered cross-functional project teams, focused around the drug development process, rather than within functional departments. Improved integration and communication of information through the use of IT is key to developing this trend further.

Building high-performance teams presents a difficult challenge, particularly in the pharmaceutical R&D context because

- bureaucratic and hierarchical organizational structures have historically hampered effective project work.
- skills of scientists in R&D have focused on scientific excellence at the expense of project management and team leadership.
- behavior of scientists from Director level to graduate entry level has prevented truly effective teamwork.
- budgeting and decision making powers on resource allocation are largely left for departmental managers with limited transfer of formal power and responsibility to project managers. Typically, people are afraid to transfer too much formal power to the project managers for fear of destabilizing the organizational matrix.
- performance management systems often do not support good teamwork across departmental interfaces and may not recognize the input from project managers. Even for team members within departments, the performance management environment does not reinforce teamwork behavior.
- the lack of effective peer groups because of geographical and departmental distance works against learning and positive competition to improve leadership and working practices.
- planning and problem solving are poor because of the lack of formal training. There is a need for simple milestones and logic-based planning tools that are easily accessible.
- increased R&D externalization means that new challenges of collaborating across companies and geographic boundaries compound the difficulties.

In addition, the nature of the activities undertaken in project teams is especially complex because

- scientific, medical and commercial knowledge is constantly changing and much of the work in R&D takes place at the leading edge.
- people with different expertise need to be integrated into the core project teams. They also need to undertake pivotal roles at interfaces between the core team and other departments and functions. The exercise of these pivotal or interface roles is difficult and often poorly executed.
- the nature of these projects is highly dynamic, affected increasingly by go/no go decisions caused by rapidly changing data. As the need for speed increases, the turnover in project terms increases with ever shorter time for teams to form and perform.
- teams are frequently split geographically with difficult communications

  – at either ends of long winding corridors,
  – at either end of large acreage sites,
  – at multiple sites in the same country, and
  – between countries.

- cultural differences, often as a result of merger/acquisition across international boundaries, highlight the issues of consistency and standards and process/reporting variations.

Cross-functional teams also need to include people beyond the direct scope of development. Traditionally, only clinicians have been involved. Cooperation with manufacturing at an early stage is becoming increasingly important to obtain faster review times combined with the possibility of new stability guidelines from the ICH (International Committee of Harmonization). Compliance with the new guidelines will require forward planning of production scale-up and methods and, thus, a need for earlier and more extensive manufacturing involvement. Traditionally, advance planning has not been a prime concern of manufacturing personnel who are more attuned to the daily issues of production runs and capacity.

B. Globalization

Globalization is a growing trend in all industries and commercial sectors as the search continues for more effective use of resources and as communication of information across geographical boundaries becomes less of a technological issue. Globalization permits organizational streamlining, leading to decreased duplication of research and production facilities and a reduction in the number of personnel required. This needs to be achieved while retaining access to the best people, the best practices, and the best facilities, regardless of location. This focus can significantly shorten the length of clinical trials. For example, a trial at the most experienced center in the world may save expensive duplications. However, in most cases, companies must distribute resources because it is not acceptable to have local trials in one center and expect the results to be accepted globally. Furthermore, within the pharmaceutical industry, a global presence is not just desirable but is, in fact, essential.

Technology is breaking these barriers down through virtualization and interactive reach. The primary issue is not technical feasibility, but how can the cultural differences between the locations be overcome.

C. Virtual Organizations

The driving force behind the development of virtual organizations, as with the drift towards globalization, is the need for more economic ways of working, thereby maximizing resources. Pharmaceutical companies are undergoing a focusing process, examining their portfolios and specifying the therapeutic areas in which to specialize. Companies are also beginning to concentrate on specific components of the drug development process and outsourcing other components where, as a means to control fixed costs, it makes more economic sense. An early example of this is the increased use of CROs (Clinical Research Organizations), whose efficiency and specialization make them a key asset for pharmaceutical companies. The logical conclusion of this development is the existence of wholly "virtual" projects where each part of the process can be outsourced—even project management (independence at the project manager level may become vital to provide neutrality for resolving cultural battles).

In recent years, the pharmaceutical industry has seen numerous acquisitions and mergers searching to extend the portfolio of products and services while continuing to focus on their own areas of specialization. When mergers or acquisitions occur, the organizations involved must become integrated and interactive as quickly as possible.

In addition, regulatory agencies are opening up, allowing ongoing, real-time reviews of data throughout the entire life cycle of a project. Already occurring, to a limited extent, for high priority drugs, this could expand to cover all drugs in development. Obviously, this will not work without changes within the pharmaceutical companies, where it is advantageous to have the time to present the data in its best light prior to any review.

Taken to its logical conclusion, the virtual organization will extend to include doctors and patients worldwide. The use of electronic case reports linked to hospital notes and of remote data entry by doctors to provide information for the clinical trials phase makes them all part of the virtual organization. As desire for outcomes data increases to justify a drug's cost and position in the market, postapproval of more sophisticated Phase IV Trials will be required.

These organizational changes will create greater amounts of information, a valuable asset in all industries, but especially in the pharmaceutical industry where the collection and use of data is fundamental in the drug development process. This information needs to be managed effectively to realize its full benefits. Information and its effective management will be the competitive weapon to take successful pharmaceutical companies into the next decade. Establishing a bank of accessible information (a data warehouse) will provide a core source of information upon which tools can be built to analyze and model future scenarios. Collecting information will become increasingly automatic, instantaneous and in a common format, making understanding and interpreting it simpler.

The major developments in IT described in section III of this chapter, together with appropriate organization and cultural change, will enable these improvements to happen.

V. FUTURE VISIONS OF PHARMACEUTICAL PROJECT MANAGEMENT

Although a lot of the changes are positive steps toward greater efficiency within pharmaceutical companies, their occurrence does not necessarily make the job of pharmaceutical project management easier. These changes create new challenges for the pharmaceutical project manager whose role must adapt, not only to cope with the changes, but to reap the most advantage from them.

The foremost concern is the resistance to change among company personnel. A high level of staff morale must be maintained alongside the introduction of new ideas, whether new organizational structures, new business practices, or new IT systems. To do this, establishing a clear operating model is essential. In many cases, the choice of operating model is irrelevant as long as it is acceptable to all staff members and has well-defined roles and responsibilities. Failure arises when no operating model has been chosen or created or when there is a hybrid of models. This lack of definition means that the path of responsibility and authority becomes confused and leads to many layers of review in the decision making process, excessive meetings, and negotiating and coordinating difficulties between teams and functions. To succeed with virtual organizations, extending this principle is even more essential to ensure that the interfaces between each element (e.g., CROs, regulatory agencies, etc.) are as equally well-defined as the interfaces between the different functions within the company.

To create high-performance teams requires, among others, the following key actions:

- unremitting focus on project objectives
- shared leadership
- all team members working at their limit
- open and intensive communication
- cohesive, compatible team membership
- a distinctive social system within the team.

When a team adopts these characteristics, its output far outstrips its previous performance. This achievement may take some effort and there is an inherent fragility about sustained high levels of performance. To make high performance the norm rather than the exception and to make the sustained level of performance robust, the change process needs to be managed, and a number of conditions need to be established (many of which can be supported and enabled by IT):

- working jointly with scientists, medics, and other personnel, considerable time and effort is required to develop the will to change and commitment to the new ways of working in teams
- formal training in specific skills
- facilitation of best practice in project settings
- peer group learning sessions
- an appropriate IT infrastructure to support and reinforce the project culture.

This does not mean that management takes care of itself. Good leadership is essential to ensure that the project progresses and does not lose its way because of too many managers and, thus, too many conflicts. To ensure this progression, first, common objectives must be established with early planning of how the objectives are to be achieved. Secondly, it is essential to communicate this focus to the team members, establishing common team values with goals aligned throughout the organization and shared by each and every team member. The promotion of a common objective requires team bonding. This bonding process across national boundaries within global teams and, similarly, within a postmerger organization, where old loyalties and different working cultures conflict, can be problematic. This is particularly true without a shared culture, heritage and training, and it is unrealistic to expect a team to function as a team until they have met in person. In this respect, the IT of today struggles to provide an adequate replacement for human interaction.

The mere existence of technological capabilities does not mean that they will be used effectively without the support, willingness, and appropriate skills of the users. Equally, information sharing capabilities mean little unless sharing is the norm. This is a difficult task because traditional organizational structures have led to fragmentation of information and knowledge (see section II of this chapter). Additionally, employees do not have the inclination, incentive, or mechanism for information sharing. For many individuals, their own unique knowledge represents their power and security, and any attempt to share that knowledge will be actively resisted. This problem will be exacerbated if the reward criteria within the organization are in opposition to the team approach.

Without successful management, these problems can expand into interdepartmental and international conflicts, creating an internal competitive focus rather than the desired process or deliverable focus. The promotion of a common objective and a productive team atmosphere is the responsibility of the project managers. They must be proactive members of the team, helping with problems and providing encouragement. Without encouragement, the team can lose its focus and motivation, leading to a decrease in productivity. It is clearly essential that the project manager is considered independent of these deliberations. This is proving difficult because project managers have their own connections and experience usually in one particular function and even one culture and location.

Continued management involvement in the process is also essential to avoid becoming excluded. Casual interaction with team members is the best way to gain "soft" information beyond the "hard" factual data supplied by any IT infrastructure. The "soft" data, for example, casual comments, judgments, and rumors are extremely important sources, and their interest and value should not be underestimated. Additionally, it is important that the virtues of intuition and judgment are recognized as valuable contributions to forming an overall balanced picture. This information is difficult to gather without some form of face-to-face contact. The project managers need to be flexible enough to continually adapt to these needs across a global (and possibly "virtual") team when they occur.

The challenge of effective information management will also intensify as greater amounts of data are produced through integration, improved channels of communication, and global/virtual teams conducting many processes simultaneously. To counteract this abundant generation of information, there need to be the right tools to permit viewpoints of information at an appropriate level, so that the information is comprehensible and relevant without excessive detail. Information overload could easily become a major problem and this will be particularly true for the project manager who resides over the whole project.

Additionally, a common language is required to describe project stages and processes between major transitions in the R&D life cycle. This will provide a valuable enabler to effective application of the principles of high-performance teamwork. This language is best established within an overall project management framework that details

- processes
- roles and responsibilities for core project team members
- key performance indicators
- skills
- information needs required to achieve high performance.

This framework needs to be readily accessible, possibly, by creating an IT-supported project team shared area or "home page," where the language and team processes can be rapidly transferred across the international organization.

Support of best practice project leadership requires regular sharing of ideas, learning, and issues within the project management peer group. Although project management must feature regularly on the agendas of international meetings of the peer group, it is also extremely important to provide an approach which allows for continuous real-time sharing of

- general project management issues including
  - planning and problem solving issues and
  - performance management issues, and
- best practice project-specific issues including
  - scientific/medical/technical issues and
  - interpersonal team dynamics issues.

Regular access to such discussion forums has, potentially, great impact across the international organization by achieving shared learning and rapid uptake of best practice. An IT-supported "home page" can support the above including performance management documentation, planning and problem solving tools, a staffing database and their own project work files. The information contained within the "home page" greatly facilitates the handover process, as projects move through the R&D life cycle, by minimizing the loss of value.

For the project manager to remain focused on the objective and ensure that it is met requires effective handling in each area of project management:

- Project planning and tracking. As a result of team empowerment and the availability of project information to each member of the project team, creating, executing, and monitoring a milestone-based project plan can become the collective responsibility of the project team, not solely of a project manager. Once established, updating of the project plan can be enabled by an integrated infrastructure feeding in relevant information.
- Business case management. A clearly defined business case showing justification for proceeding with a drug development project must be created, and more importantly, reviewed and updated regularly. Integration and improved communication infrastructures will aid this process, providing timely information and facilitating easier tracking of key drivers. This will enable making important decisions earlier and with greater confidence rather than relying solely on "gut feelings." Moreover, the availability of information to all members of the project team means that development opportunities can be assessed from many perspectives by a multiskilled team. This should include greater marketing input and scientific assessment to ensure that products are developed with the correct indications and that priorities between projects are correctly set.
  Technology can also help with reuse by collecting and synthesizing historical information to provide benchmarking for future projects. Even external factors can be assessed more effectively by tracking them with such a framework. Improved business case management can reduce cost and lead time significantly by weeding out marginal products.
- Resource management/capacity planning. Greater internal visibility of information through integration allows improved assessment of

present resource requirements and availability. In addition, access to a catalogue of data from previous drug development projects improves forecasting predictions in resource management and allocation. The decision to outsource because internal resources are lacking will become clearer (and easier outsourcing will be enabled by integration and virtualization).

- Portfolio management. Improving cultural alignment by establishing consistent standards across projects will facilitate more informed portfolio management. Thus, the impact of resource needs, costs and timescales of individual projects on other concurrent projects will be clearer. This clarity is vital as globalization and the use of external organizations increases.

In conclusion, the pharmaceutical industry will inevitably change, not through technological innovations but rather in response to the many pressures it faces. However, it is not true that technology is a limiting factor in industry progress. The technology is available today, but it requires people and processes and management to embrace it ("the future is already here, it is just unevenly distributed").

Although technology will facilitate aspects of the project management function, it is merely a tool which cannot provide miracle solutions. Paradoxically, IT systems can often increase, rather than reduce, the responsibilities of those who work with them ("ignorance is bliss").

In general, pharmaceutical project management must assume a more integral and empowered role within the drug development process, valued as a function/skill by all project team members, rather than being purely reactive and effectively powerless.

The development of IT capabilities coupled with effective project management will bring many benefits to pharmaceutical companies. This is essential for companies to survive and prosper in the changing industrial environment.

Index